Also by Mark Hyman, M.D.

UltraMetabolism

The UltraSimple Diet

Ultraprevention (with Mark Liponis, M.D.)

The Detox Box

The 5 Forces of Wellness

Nutrigenomics

The

UltraMetabolism

Cookbook

**200 Delicious Recipes That
Will Turn on Your Fat-Burning DNA**

Mark Hyman, M.D.

Recipes by Donna Boland

Scribner
New York   London   Toronto   Sydney

This publication contains the opinions and ideas of the author. It is intended to provide helpful and in-formative material on the subjects addressed in the publication. It is sold with the understanding that the author and publisher are not engaged in rendering medical, health, psychological, or any other kind of personal professional services in the book. If the reader requires personal medical, health, or other assis-tance or advice, a competent professional should be consulted.

The author and publisher specifically disclaim all responsibility for any liability, loss, or risk, personal or otherwise, that is incurred as a consequence, directly or indirectly, of the use and application of any of the contents of this book.

 Scribner
A Division of Simon & Schuster, Inc.
1230 Avenue of the Americas
New York, NY 10020

First Scribner hardcover edition November 2007

SCRIBNER and design are trademarks of Macmillan Library Reference USA, Inc.,
used under license by Simon & Schuster, the publisher of this work.

For information about special discounts for bulk purchases,
please contact Simon & Schuster Special Sales at 1-800-456-6798
or business@simonandschuster.com

Designed by Ruth Lee-Mui

Manufactured in the United States of America

10   9   8   7   6   5   4   3   2

Library of Congress Cataloging-in-Publication Data

Hyman, Mark, 1959–
    The ultrametabolism cookbook : 200 easy to make delicious recipes that will turn on your fat
burning DNA / Mark Hyman. — 1st Scribner hardcover ed.
        p.   cm.
    1. Weight loss.   Reducing diets—Recipes.   3. Metabolism.   4. Nutrition.
I. Title.

RM222.2.H966   2007
641.5'63—dc22   2007029723

ISBN-13: 978-1-4165-4959-8
ISBN-10:   1-4165-4959-5

CONTENTS

LIST OF RECIPES

PHASE I

PHASE II

Vinaigrettes, Sauces, and Dressings

A PERSONAL NOTE ON MY EXPERIENCES WITH FOOD

Let food be thy medicine and medicine be thy food.

——HIPPOCRATES

Whole Food, Real Food: Food as Medicine

Sitting at my friend's home in the Umbrian countryside, looking out over the olive orchard and fields of sunflowers, having just had a home-cooked meal prepared by Simonetta, it was clear to me why so many Italians are thin and happy. Family, friends, and fresh, whole foods are all interwoven into the pleasure of being alive.

The meal was served on a long wooden table, set with beautiful ceramic plates painted with sunflowers. Simonetta made light chicken meatballs with a fresh tomato sauce, accompanied by an arugula and radicchio salad and a side salad of vine-ripened, freshly picked garden tomatoes, fresh basil, roasted peppers, and grilled eggplant, drizzled with fresh extra-virgin olive oil made from the olive trees surrounding the old stone farmhouse in which we dined.

The food in this ancient countryside is grown and prepared locally. A meal from a box or can is a strange notion in these hills; food made with labels a hard thing to find. No one here is on a diet. Food is a source of pleasure, not anxiety. How far so many of us have come from this simple way of preparing, eating, and enjoying real, whole, fresh foods!

Looking back on my life, I realize how important whole foods have been to me since a very early age. I was born in Barcelona and spent my first four years there, discovering the smells of the marketplace and freshly prepared Catalan dishes. My mother always had a small garden and since the age of eighteen, I've grown my own vegetables. I inherited the love of fresh food and cooking from my mother, and the joy of eating from my father. Bringing together family and friends and preparing nourishing, delicious meals from whole, fresh ingredients is one of my life's greatest pleasures.

Now, as a doctor specializing in nutritional medicine, I realize how fundamentally important this simple pleasure is. Our bodies and souls thrive on fresh, whole real food. To eat well is to be healthy. Food *is* medicine. It cures us.

Despite how simple this seems, it is the cure for most of our chronic diseases and the obesity epidemic. It is one of the keys to living a fulfilling and vitally healthy life in this modern age, just as it was millennia ago in the Mediterranean countryside.

What I am asking you to do is eat foods that come from the earth, not from a box or can or prepared by food scientists in a factory. These factory-processed foods are unrecognizable by our genes and our cells, which respond the best they can. They accommodate to these foods by making us sick.

You can make a different choice. This book will help you take advantage of ancient cultural wisdom about food and modern nutritional science. Your cells, your genes, and your soul will thank you.

The

UltraMetabolism

Cookbook

ULTRAMETABOLISM: A REVOLUTION IN FOOD AND MEDICINE

Food is our source of nourishment. It is also a source of pleasure, and eating is a way of celebrating with family and friends. Yet for many of us, food has become an enemy—a source of confusion, bewilderment, frustration, and even anger.

Most of us know that the way we eat does not help us thrive. In fact, over two-thirds of Americans struggle with their weight. In addition, many of us worry that what we eat will increase our risk of heart disease, cancer, diabetes, and dementia. We battle cravings and desires that no longer match our body's true needs . . . and we know it. Yet we are stuck in an awful cycle, trapped by patterns of eating we don't know how to escape.

UltraMetabolism and this cookbook are based on principles that will help you reverse that downward spiral and become friends with food once again, so it can become a source of nourishment and healing and the key to achieving UltraWellness—lifelong health and vitality.

I decided to create this cookbook because of the many requests I received for more delicious recipes like the ones originally included in *UltraMetabolism: The Simple Plan for Automatic Weight Loss*. We worked diligently to put together a re-markable set of recipes that have been tested relentlessly by both professional chefs and everyday folks to ensure they are easy to make, delicious, and, most important, follow the exact nutritional guidelines I described in *UltraMetabolism*, which I will review for you a bit later.

I've designed this cookbook to be as user-friendly as possible—all of the recipes are organized so you know specifically in which phase of the Ultra-Metabolism program you can use them, and they are all tagged so you can quickly determine whether a particular recipe contains something you might be allergic to, whether that's wheat, dairy, eggs, or any other common allergen.

IMPORTANT: Before reading further, please go to http://www.ultrameta bolismcookbook.com/guide and download The UltraMetabolism Cookbook Companion Guide, which contains dozens of helpful tips and resources to make cooking easier, quicker, and more delicious.

What Is UltraMetabolism?

UltraMetabolism: The Simple Plan for Automatic Weight Loss gave many the chance to know what it's like to feel good again—to have more energy, to be free from many chronic symptoms, and to lose weight automatically without suffering. UltraMetabolism is a program based on eating in harmony with our genes, eating the real, whole foods on which our bodies were designed to function—not the processed, altered, alien food devoid of nutrients and nourishment that, unfortunately, most of us eat today.

One of the things that twenty years of practicing medicine has taught me is this: The same things that make us sick also make us fat. By dealing with the underlying causes of disease—what we eat, how we move our bodies (or don't), and how we deal with stress—we can effectively address at least 80 to 90 percent of all illness, as well as the current obesity epidemic.

However, nutrition is not traditionally considered a part of medicine (except that it provides the energy needs of the body). Through no fault of their own, most physicians are nutritionally illiterate, because they received little or no nutrition education in their medical training.

Yet food is the most powerful tool we have to promote good health and treat disease. It is the single best medicine in my medical tool kit. Conversely, food can also cause disease and suffering. Food is both healer and slayer.

I didn't start out in medicine with this knowledge about the power of food. I had to learn the hard way, from over twenty years of treating patients and testing to see precisely what worked and what didn't, to understand that conventional methods really didn't work that well. The real secret, I found, was to work with the nutritional intelligence inherent in whole, real foods to help heal the body.

The science of nutrition has advanced far beyond what the average person hears about in the media or from health care practitioners. Consensus among scientists and researchers about what constitutes a healthy diet actually does exist. Unfortunately, we don't hear about this research because the food industry and the government encourage confusion and the consumption of foods that feed profit, not health.

It often takes up to twenty years for scientific findings like these to be integrated into common medical practice. But the information we need about how important proper nutrition is for the human body is available *right now*. I wrote *UltraMetabolism* to give you the opportunity to take advantage of this wealth of information today instead of waiting for the medical industry to catch up with modern research. In it, I give a step-by-step program for rebalancing the seven key systems in the body that control health and weight loss. I explain how eating a real, whole-foods diet is the single most important factor for losing weight and regaining your health.

This cookbook is an extension of that program. It is based on the collective nutritional intelligence of the last three decades of research. It may not only help you lose weight and maintain weight loss, but may also help you resolve many chronic health problems that conventional medicine does not adequately address.

There is no reason to wait for nutritional science to become common knowledge. You can take advantage of my hard-won experience as a medical practitioner and decades of research in nutritional science to heal your body and nourish your soul, to become friends with food once again, and to make eating an *enjoyable* experience.

That is what this cookbook is designed to help you do. The recipes are built on the same principles that made *UltraMetabolism* such a powerful experience for so many. All you have to do is follow the recipes, and you are already on your way to becoming thin and healthy.

But to take full advantage of this cookbook and the science that *UltraMetabolism* is based on, you need to have some background in the key principles that make the program work.

Again, remember to download the companion guide to this cookbook at http://www.ultrametabolismcookbook.com/guide to get access to extra tips, tricks, and techniques on shopping for, preparing, and cooking your meals.

The Seven Keys to UltraMetabolism

The seven keys described in *UltraMetabolism* are part of the seven keys to health and well-being—to what I call UltraWellness, which is nothing short of lifelong health and vitality. They are based on a revolutionary new understanding of how the body works called Functional Medicine.

This new science teaches us that what you eat directly affects the causes of disease, among which are impaired appetite regulation, digestive function, stress, inflammation, oxidative stress (or rusting), impaired energy metabolism, hormone and neurotransmitter imbalances, and inadequate detoxification. The seven keys to UltraMetabolism are based on the seven roots of illness, which are also the seven keys to UltraWellness.

When you attack illness and weight gain at the root by getting these systems back into balance, you transform what was plaguing you into an ally on your quest for vital health and weight loss. You release yourself from the trap that has been keeping you sick and fat for so long.

You can deal with these seven factors *effortlessly* by choosing foods that heal rather than harm. When you do, you will begin a lifetime of health and automatic weight loss. The ingredients and foods included in the recipes here help the body function as it was designed to and correct many of the underlying causes of disease—the imbalances in these keys.

To understand how this works, you need to understand a bit about the keys themselves. The seven keys to UltraMetabolism are:

1. Control your appetite
2. Subdue stress

3. Cool the fire of inflammation
4. Prevent oxidative stress or "rust"
5. Turn calories into energy
6. Fortify your thyroid
7. Love your liver

These seven keys all work together to open the door to vitality, health, and successful long-term weight loss. They are the keys to reversing disease, being set free of chronic symptoms, and creating optimal health. The following is a very brief summary of each of these keys. For a more detailed look, I strongly encourage you to read *UltraMetabolism: The Simple Plan for Automatic Weight Loss*. You can access a sneak preview of the book by going to http://www.ultrametabolismcook book.com/um-preview.

Key #1: Control Your Appetite

The first key is to understand how your brain, gut, and fat cells communicate with one another through hormones and brain messenger chemicals to tell you whether or not you need food and to compel you to eat. When they are working properly, they are an elegant machine pinpointing when you need energy and asking you to consume calories to obtain that energy. When they go haywire—and there are *many* ways for them to go haywire in our current eating climate—they cause you to eat when you don't need to, contributing to weight gain and almost every other health problem we face.

Key #2: Subdue Stress

The second key is to understand how stress makes you fat and how to overcome its effects. Under any physical or psychological stress, the body is designed to protect itself. It stores calories and conserves weight (you might need that energy reserve to run from a predator). It pumps hormones into your system that increase blood fats, sugar, and insulin to prepare you for fight or flight. Without eating more or exercising less, stress alone will cause weight gain.

Key #3: Cool the Fire of Inflammation

The third key is controlling inflammation, a hidden force behind weight gain and disease. Being overweight promotes inflammation and inflammation promotes obesity in a terrible, vicious cycle. More than half of Americans are inflamed, and most of them don't know it.

Key #4: Prevent Oxidative Stress or "Rust"

The fourth key is preventing cellular "rust" that interferes with metabolism, contributes to weight gain and aging, and causes inflammation. Free radicals are oxygen molecules that run around your body stealing electrons from other molecules. The molecule that loses an electron is damaged, or oxidized. Oxidized tissues and cells don't function normally. The process results in damaged DNA, damaged cell membranes, stiff arteries that look like rusted pipes, and wrinkles.

Key #5: Turn Calories into Energy

The fifth key is learning how to turbocharge your metabolic engine to more efficiently turn calories into energy. Your ability to burn calories is dependent on the health, number, and efficiency of your mitochondria, the little powerhouses that produce energy in every cell. You can reverse the damage that's been done to your mitochondria and turn up your metabolic fire if you know how.

Key #6: Fortify Your Thyroid

The sixth key is making sure your thyroid, the master metabolism hormone, is working optimally. Twenty percent of all women and about ten percent of men have a sluggish thyroid, slowing their metabolism; half of them are undiagnosed. Many of those who are diagnosed are not treated optimally, making matters worse.

Key #7: Love Your Liver

The seventh key is detoxifying your liver so it will properly metabolize sugars and fats. Toxins from within our bodies and toxins from our environment both contribute to obesity. Getting rid of toxins and boosting your natural detoxification system is an essential component of long-term weight loss and a healthy metabolism.

The single biggest factor that impacts each of these keys is the food you eat. By eating a whole-foods diet, like the one presented in this cookbook, you will rebalance these key systems, and begin losing weight and regaining your health automatically.

The secret lies in a revolutionary new science, one that isn't largely known by the mainstream medical community but contains the scientific research necessary to heal many of the diseases people in our society suffer from, as well as the obesity epidemic. This science is called *nutrigenomics*.

Nutrigenomics: The Science Behind UltraMetabolism

The philosophy of UltraMetabolism is based on the notion that you can change your genes by what you eat. Though your genetic code is fixed when you are born, the genes that get turned on or off are influenced by many factors, the most important of which is food. This is the new science of nutrigenomics—or how nutrients influence which genes are expressed, which in turn controls your health and your weight.

When people first hear about this concept, questions immediately arise. How does food influence your genes? Aren't they fixed? Aren't they responsible for things like determining the color of your eyes and hair? How can you change your genes? And what influence does that have on your weight and health?

Let me offer some answers.

Your DNA isn't quite as rigid and fixed as you think. Think of your DNA as though it were the hardware inside a computer—no matter what software you load onto your computer, this hardware doesn't change. But by loading different types of software, whether a word processing program, a graphic design program, or an e-mail program, you can get your computer to perform different functions.

In the same way, you can load "software" into your body and get it to perform different functions by providing it with different types of information. This information comes in the form of the food that you choose to consume. Depending on what you eat, different types of your DNA hardware are expressed or turned on.

In fact, food is the most important factor that controls how your genes—your hardware—are expressed or used. Food controls parts of your genetic functioning that create health or promote disease. Whole foods turn on the health and weight-loss genes. Processed foods, high in sugar and trans fats, turn on the disease and weight-gain genes.

The most powerful tool you have to change how your genes function is your fork.

The foods and ingredients that make up *The UltraMetabolism Cookbook* are included because they turn on the genes that help you control your appetite and improve your digestive function, control inflammation, improve detoxification, balance your hormones, reduce oxidative stress or rusting, balance the stress response, and enhance thyroid function.

They are simple, real, whole, nourishing foods that give your body the ingredients it needs to thrive. This is the way to help your cells and your soul become fully alive.

One of the keys to turning on genes that cause you to lose weight lies in the *phytonutrient* content of the foods you eat. Plant foods and human beings co-evolved. We are designed to thrive on the chemicals that plants provide us with. These chemicals are the hidden medicine in the food we eat, and without them our health deteriorates. To understand why the seven keys to UltraMetabolism are so powerful, you need to understand what phytonutrients are.

Phytonutrients: Food's Hidden Medicine

Some of the most potent compounds in foods are the color pigments found in fruits and vegetables. These are called phytochemicals or phytonutrients. Our bodies have evolved to use these compounds to turn on genes that promote health and reverse disease.

For example, there are the *anthocyanidins* in cherries that control inflammation, the *glucosinolates* in broccoli that help your body detoxify environmental toxins, the *catechins* in green tea that boost metabolism and help prevent cancer, and the *polysaccharides* in shiitake mushrooms that boost immunity.

These phytonutrients were not created for our benefit. The plants' "design" was certainly not to help us prevent disease. Plants developed these phytonutrients to protect themselves from infection, stress, and other hardships; in other words, to ensure their survival.

Organic plants have a harder time of things and are under more stress than crops grown in large monocultures (where there is only one crop, for example corn, grown on an entire field), supported by petrochemical nitrogen fertilizers and protected from danger by pesticides and herbicides. Organic plants have to survive a harsher environment.

Put another way, plants grown organically have had to sink or swim, to develop their own defenses against their natural enemies, and the defenses they have grown are these very phytonutrients. Because they have grown in a more challenging environment, they produce more potent phytochemicals.

Conventionally grown plants that have the help of fertilizers, pesticides, and herbicides naturally don't have to work as hard and therefore produce fewer phytonutrients. Therefore, when you eat conventionally grown plants, you miss out on some of the powerful benefits of these phytonutrients.★ This is one of the reasons it's good to choose organic food whenever possible. You will get more phytonutrients out of organic food than conventionally grown plants, due to the fact that these plants had to fight harder to survive.

These phytonutrients are critically important for us, because our bodies are generally lazy (or, put another way, magnificently efficient). When it comes to any extra biochemical effort, they have evolved to use the phytonutrients found in plants to protect us against disease. For example, the human body does not

★ Heaton and Shane, 2001. *Organic Farming Food Quality and Human Health*. The Soil Association. Bristol, UK.

produce vitamin C on its own, though many other species do. The reason? We can easily get it from the foods we eat, so we don't *have* to produce it on our own.

So, as you can see, over the many millions of years of evolution, we've grown dependent on plants as a source for these powerful phytonutrients to defend our bodies. Let's look at some of the health benefits of these healing chemicals.

Foods and Phytonutrients: Health Benefits

Healing chemicals in foods may in the end be more important than the protein, fat, carbohydrates, vitamins, and minerals they contain. Practically the only thing everyone agrees about in nutrition is that eating five to nine servings of fruits and vegetables a day can reduce your risk from almost every known disease of our "modern" civilization, including heart disease, stroke, Alzheimer's, and cancer.

You certainly have heard that soy lowers cholesterol, or that broccoli helps prevent cancer, or that tomatoes help prevent prostate cancer. But phytonutrients exist in a vast array of plant foods, and eating a wide variety of fruits and vegetables is one of the best ways to acquire the nutrients you need to protect yourself from illness and help you lose weight.

Many of us fall into monotony in our vegetable choices. To maximize the benefit of these healing foods, choose from the incredibly rich variety of colorful fruits and vegetables. Think color! Try something different!

The following guidelines will help you make the most of phytonutrients.

Guidelines for Maximizing Phytonutrient Intake

Choose from the following varieties of fruits and vegetables:

- ❖ **Red, yellow, and orange fruits and vegetables** (tomatoes, red peppers, mangoes, papaya, pineapple, chili peppers, sweet potatoes, winter squash, cantaloupe, peaches, carrots, apricots). These contain an abundance of antioxidants including the carotenoids lutein and lycopene, which can help prevent macular degeneration and prostate and other cancers. They also contain quercitin, which can help reduce inflammation and allergy.

- **Dark green leafy vegetables** (kale, collard greens, spinach, dandelion greens, mustard greens). These contain antioxidants and carotenoids that help protect against aging, heart disease, and cancer. They also contain magnesium and folate, two critical nutrients in which many people are deficient.

- **Dark blue, purple, or red fruits and vegetables** (blueberries, blackberries, cherries, plums, beets, red onions, purple grapes, red cabbage, radicchio). In addition to vitamins and minerals, these are rich sources of antioxidants such as the phenols, ellagic acid, and anthocyanoside, as well as terpenes that boost immune function and help fight cancer. Cherries have very powerful anti-inflammatory proanthocyanidins.

- **Cruciferous vegetables** (broccoli, cabbage, kale, collards, kohlrabi, brussel sprouts, bok choy, Chinese broccoli). These are rich sources of isothiocyanates and indoles, which have been shown to increase liver detoxification and prevent cancer.

- **Allium vegetables** (garlic, onions, leeks, shallots). These contain an abundance of health-promoting properties including organosulfur compounds, critical for detoxification of toxic chemicals. They also contain phenols like quercitin, which has powerful antimicrobial and anti-inflammatory compounds. In addition, garlic can lower blood pressure, thin the blood, lower cholesterol, and treat infections.

- **Citrus fruits** (lemons, limes, oranges, grapefruit). These contain limonene, a terpene, which can help with liver detoxification and can prevent cancer and heart disease. They are also rich in bioflavinoids, including hesperedin, that are very anti-inflammatory and anti-carcinogenic, as well as rich in carotenoids such as lycopene and lutein.

- **Flaxseed.** These seeds are rich sources of lignans, which have very important hormone-modulating effects that can prevent breast cancer and help with hormonal disorders. They also promote healthy gut bacterial flora and can reduce menopausal symptoms.

- **Legumes** (or beans). These contain all sorts of healing chemicals including saponins, compounds that reduce the risk of heart disease and cancer and boost immunity. The fiber also helps promote healthy gut ecology, and certain compounds called protease inhibitors may prevent cancer.

- ⁘ **Soybeans and soy products.** These contain daidzein, genistein, and a protease inhibitor called BBI that protects against cancer and lowers cholesterol.

- ⁘ **Tea** (mostly green). Green tea contains epigallactocatechins that boost liver detoxification, reduce cholesterol, reduce inflammation, and can help prevent cancer and heart disease. It is also thermogenic, and may help increase metabolism and promote weight loss.

- ⁘ **Sea vegetables** (kelp, dulse, kombu, hijiki, arame). Besides containing higher levels of more minerals, including iodine, than any other food, they are rich sources of carotenoids and phenols such as ellagic acid that can prevent cancer.

- ⁘ **Spices.** Turmeric (found in curries) contains curcumin, a potent anti-inflammatory, anti-oxidant, and booster of liver detoxification that protects against environmental pollution. Rosemary contains ursolic acid, a very potent anti-inflammatory chemical. Purple sage contains anti-inflammatory compounds. These are just a few among many examples of healing spices.

Table 1-1 is a quick reference for just a few of the more powerful plant foods, the phytonutrients they contain, and the health benefits that result. It is not comprehensive—almost *all* plant foods contain important chemicals—but it should expand your understanding of just how important these foods are.

It is not important to remember every chemical in every food. Just remember to choose foods as if you were choosing paints to create a beautiful Monet or Matisse landscape. Choose a variety of bright colors: yellows, oranges, reds, purple, and greens.

UltraMetabolism and the recipes in this cookbook are created around these powerful phytonutrients. They will help you leverage the power of plant foods so you can use phytonutrients to help you lose weight.

Table 1-1: Phytonutrients in Food

Food	Type of Phytonutrients	Health Benefits
Green tea	Catechins	Anti-inflammatory, detoxifying, prevents cancer
Tomatoes	Lycopene	Antioxidant, prevents cancer
Broccoli	Glucosinolates	Increases detoxification
Cherries	Proanthocyanidins	Anti-inflammatory
Turmeric	Curcuminoids	Anti-inflammatory, antioxidant, prevents cancer and dementia
Shiitake mushrooms	Polysaccharides	Boost immune system and prevent cancer
Ginger	Gingerols	Anti-inflammatory
Citrus peels	Limonene and terpenoids	Enhance detoxification
Garlic	Organosulfur compounds and phenols	Boosts immune system, antimicrobial, anti-inflammatory, detoxifying
Soy	Isoflavones	Prevents cancer, lowers cholesterol, reduces inflammation
Flaxseed	Lignans	Prevents cancer, lower cholesterol
Pomegranates	Ellagitannin	Lower blood pressure and prevent and even reverse heart disease, prevent cancer by reducing DNA damage, reduce inflammation

Phytonutrients are not the only benefit of a well-balanced, whole-foods diet that includes lots of plant foods. When you eat the UltraMetabolism way, you learn to take advantage of these "good" carbohydrates by balancing your *glycemic load*.

Glycemic Load: The Secret to Health Is Balancing Your Blood Sugar

One of the surprising truths I unveiled in *UltraMetabolism* is that carbohydrates (contrary to popular belief) are the most important nutrient in your diet. Without them, you quickly become malnourished and your health declines, because they contain nearly all the vitamins, minerals, fiber, and phytonutrients you need to thrive.

Remember, carbohydrates are not just bread, spaghetti, and potatoes—they include fruits, vegetables, whole grains, beans, nuts, and seeds. Because many popular diets on the market defame carbohydrates, a lot of people have the mistaken impression that carbohydrates consist only of highly processed foods that are built on what I call "the white menace"—white flour, white sugar, or some variant of these. These are indeed "bad" carbs, but they do not account for *all* carbs, some of which are critically important for your health.

As you know from *UltraMetabolism*, there is a big difference between the highly processed carbs that count for most of the real estate in your local supermarket and whole, unprocessed carbs. To help you identify the difference between "good" carbs and "bad" carbs, I suggest you replace all the old (and abundant) terminology surrounding carbohydrates with two simple concepts:

- Glycemic Load (GL)
- Phytonutrient Index (PI)

We define the *glycemic load* of a food or meal as the total effect that food or meal has on your blood sugar. The food or meals you eat can have either a *high glycemic load* or a *low glycemic load*.

A high glycemic load means carbohydrates in the food you eat are absorbed by your body rapidly, hence they raise your blood sugar rapidly. Foods or meals that have a low glycemic load do just the opposite—they make your body work to absorb the sugar, so your blood sugar goes up more slowly.

There are a number of reasons it's important that your blood sugar rises and

falls in a slow and smooth arc. If it doesn't, the sophisticated web of hormones and chemicals that control your metabolism (including and perhaps most importantly insulin) falls into chaos, sending your metabolism (not to mention your appetite) out of balance. When this happens, all kinds of health problems ensue, including weight gain, obesity, and diabetes.

There are many factors that determine the glycemic load of the foods you eat, including their fat, carbohydrate, fiber, and protein content. I won't explain how all of these factors affect glycemic load here. For a more detailed discussion, read *UltraMetabolism*, a free sneak preview of which can be found at http://www .ultrametabolismcookbook.com/um-preview.

Generally it is most effective to look at the glycemic load of an entire meal, instead of looking at it on a food-by-food basis. The composition of your meals is more important than the single foods you eat. This is because even foods with the highest glycemic loads can be offset by other foods with lower glycemic loads. For example, if you add enough fiber to foods with very high glycemic load, like cola, you can make them low-glycemic-load foods. (Don't get the wrong impression. I'm not giving you an excuse to drink soda!)

This means the meals you compose should consist primarily of low-glycemic-load foods. Not *all* of the foods you eat have to be low glycemic load, but *most* of them should be.

The *phytonutrient index* defines how many phytonutrients are in a given food. I have already given you a comprehensive definition of phytonutrients. With this information, understanding the index is simple: The more phytonutrients in a given food, the higher it lies on the phytonutrient index.

When it comes to carbohydrates, the nutritional secret of *UltraMetabolism* is simple:

Eat foods with a low glycemic load (GL) and high phytonutrient index (PI).

To help you remember what this means, here is a list of low-GL/high-PI foods:

+ Vegetables
+ Fruits

- Beans
- Whole grains
- Nuts
- Seeds
- Unrefined, expeller-pressed oils (extra-virgin olive oil, coconut oil, etc.)
- Teas
- Herbs and spices

Keep in mind that animal protein falls in a separate category because it does not have phytonutrients, so you can't choose the animal protein you eat based on these standards.

If you can remember to eat foods with a low GL and a high PI, you can forget about ALL the other terms used to define and describe carbohydrates.

Eating for Health and Pleasure: Food as Healer/Food as Slayer

I find it odd that our palate has adapted to flavorless, packaged foods designed in food laboratories. These foods become like drugs—we need more and more of them to keep us satisfied and the satisfaction decreases every time we use them.

Those who eat junk food, processed food, or packaged foods with a high GL and a low PI that are high in sugar, trans fats, and food additives actually eat more food (and calories) than people who consume real, whole, fresh foods.

These unhealthful foods, like heroin, are addictive. They have fewer nutrients, so we crave (and eat) more food to try to satisfy our starving cells. We feel good only while eating them; shortly thereafter we revert to feeling foggy, tired, bloated, sluggish, and numb. The pleasure we get from them is fleeting and false.

In fact, when we eat nutritionally depleted foods we crave more. Children who are iron deficient will eat dirt, a condition known as pica, in an attempt to get what their body needs. Those who eat a nutritionally deficient diet will consume more of those foods in the vain attempt to get more nutrients. Unfortunately, that will never happen, so they just eat more and more.

It is no surprise that the food that makes us fat also makes us sick.

On the other hand, if we change our diet to real, whole, fresh foods, not only will we learn to enjoy the fruits (and vegetables) of the earth, but we will also reconstitute our bodies with the right ingredients and nourish our cells so that health returns to us naturally and automatically. The pleasures of good food and good health are inevitably intertwined. Feeling good and eating well go together.

Many of us must go through a short period of withdrawal (two to three days) from our out-of-control, addictive eating patterns based on processed, nutritionally depleted foods while we learn to prepare and taste real food. However, once we do that, we remember what it feels like to feel good again—to have a body that naturally regulates its appetite and desires.

Once you get a taste for how good you can really feel, you'll realize how bad you actually felt and you'll never want to go back to your old ways of eating.

That is what *UltraMetabolism* and *The UltraMetabolism Cookbook* will help you do.

HOW ULTRAMETABOLISM WORKS: A QUICK REVIEW OF THE EIGHT-WEEK PROGRAM FOR SIMPLE, AUTOMATIC WEIGHT LOSS AND HEALTH

UltraMetabolism is a two-phase program with a one-week preparation phase. The first phase lasts three weeks and helps you resolve metabolic problems. It involves a period of cleansing and renewal through detoxification. During this time you may feel more energetic, lose weight, relieve many chronic health problems, and improve energy, memory, digestion, sleep, and allergies.

The second phase starts with a four-week introductory period, but it actually lasts a lifetime. It will help you live in harmony with your genes and rebalance your hormones, immune system, and energy metabolism and achieve Ultra-Wellness—lifelong health and vitality.

You will finally have the owner's manual for your body you have always wanted. Following this eating plan is the heart of the program; doing this will help you lose weight and get healthy.

Food as Medicine

In the Chinese language, the word for eating is comprised of the characters for "eat rice," or *chi fan*. The characters for "take medicine" are *chi yao*. In Chinese culture, eating food and eating medicine are synonymous. Food is medicine.

Modern science also teaches us to use food as medicine. The delicious, simple, nourishing menus in *UltraMetabolism* and in this cookbook use real, traditional, whole foods and were created on principles derived from the current collective scientific wisdom, as well as nutritional knowledge of our evolutionary diets. This is the diet on which our bodies were designed to thrive.

The recipes you will find here have been designed to fit into a busy life. Many have short preparation and cooking times so you can prepare a delicious and healthy meal on a limited schedule. But keep in mind that even the fastest meals cannot be made without some forethought and organization.

Most of us don't plan our meals. Then we suddenly end up in an alarm state, hungry and on the hunt. We have become a nation of drive-by eaters. This is the worst way to eat if you want to get healthy and lose weight.

You are going to have to put some effort into achieving your goals. Turning your metabolism into an UltraMetabolism will require planning, shopping, and preparation. The energy you put into creating these wonderful dishes will pay off.

In addition, you will need to be open-minded. You are going to discover new ingredients that offer potent nutritional benefits and wonderful flavors, and help create a healthy metabolism. Some of these ingredients won't be familiar to you. Remember, we live in a culture that has convinced us that unhealthy foods are good for us.

Some of the familiar has to be abandoned to rebuild a diet that is healthy and will help you lose weight. Be open to trying new things. I think you will find them quite delicious. And I am sure you will find they give you more energy and make you feel better than many of the foods you were eating before.

Learning to incorporate these new foods into your diet and figuring out where to find them and how to prepare them takes time. Be patient. Food has become the enemy for many. Don't let these new foods be your enemy.

It is time now to make friends, to celebrate food, and to discover something new. Despite the cultural and marketing pressures that surround us, eating well is not impossible. Food is an adventure down the road to your birthright—feeling fabulous and fit.

When you follow the program, food will once again become a friend, a source of nourishment, a pleasure to eat, and a delight to share with friends and family. We all have a fit person inside of us waiting to emerge.

We all can fit into our jeans if we learn how to fit into our genes by feeding them what they deserve. UltraMetabolism will teach you how to do that.

The Principles of Eating to Create an UltraMetabolism

The two-phase UltraMetabolism plan was designed to help you reach and maintain a healthy weight and metabolism for life. It is not meant to be a diet, but a way of life.

It is not a low-fat, low-carb, or calorie-restricted diet, but a program meant to help you relearn the joy of eating real food, slow food, and less food, based on traditional diets that have kept us free from degenerative disease and obesity for millennia—much like the Mediterranean and Asian diets on which it is largely based. Food should nourish our palates, our bodies, and our souls. These are not mutually exclusive.

In short, the program is based on a handful of simple, scientifically founded principles that tell us how we should eat for maximum health. These concepts are derived from extensive medical research and years of clinical practice, and while they may need to be customized for the individual, they form the basic blueprint for healthy eating.

In this book, these principles have been translated into menus and recipes that are easy to prepare from commonly found ingredients that are delicious, pleasing, and satisfying.

As long as you stick to the following principles (which are the core concepts upon which *UltraMetabolism* is based), you will be able to maintain your health and your desired weight for life.

I have expanded on some of these principles below, and you will find a complete outline of each of them in *UltraMetabolism: The Simple Plan for Automatic Weight Loss.*

20 PRINCIPLES OF A HEALTHY DIET

1. Low-glycemic-load meals
2. Combination of protein, fat, and carbohydrates to reduce glycemic load
3. High fiber—30 to 50 grams a day
4. Increased omega-3 fatty acids, monounsaturated fats
5. Colorful diversity of low-glycemic vegetables and fruits
6. Anti-inflammatory foods
7. Detoxifying foods
8. Antioxidant foods
9. Increased intake of nuts, seeds, and legumes
10. Whole soy foods
11. Lean animal protein
12. Whole grains (minimal flours)
13. Minimize or eliminate refined flours and sugars
14. Little caffeine
15. No artificial sweeteners or high-fructose corn syrup
16. No trans fats and few saturated fats (less than 5 percent of calories)
17. Greater meal frequency
18. Lower meal quantity
19. Eating breakfast
20. Not eating two to three hours before bed

I have expanded on some of these principles below, and you will find a complete outline of each of them in *UltraMetabolism: The Simple Plan for Automatic Weight Loss.*

UltraMetabolism: Some Important General Guidelines

Meal Timing

✣ **Include protein for breakfast** every day, such as whole omega-3 eggs, (soy or rice) protein shakes, and nut butters.

✣ **Eat something every four hours** to keep your insulin and glucose levels normal.

✣ **Eat a small nutrient-dense protein snack** in the morning and afternoon, such as a handful of almonds.

✣ **Avoid eating two to three hours before bed when possible**. Eating before bed interferes with sleep, but, more important, your body is in storage mode when sleeping—so you gain weight.

Meal Composition

✣ **Controlling the glycemic load** of your meals is very important. You can do this by combining adequate protein, fats, and whole-food carbohydrates from vegetables, legumes, nuts, seeds, and fruit at every meal or snack. It is most important to avoid eating quickly absorbed carbohydrates alone, as they raise your sugar and insulin levels.

Choose from a Variety of the Following Foods

✣ Choose **organic produce and animal products** whenever possible.

✣ Cold-water **fish** such as salmon, halibut, and sable contain an abundance of **beneficial essential fatty acids**—omega-3 oils that reduce inflammation. Canned wild salmon is a great emergency food.

✣ Eat high-quality **protein**, such as fish, especially fatty, cold-water fish like salmon, sable, small halibut, herring, and sardines; shellfish.

✣ Eat **omega-3 eggs**—up to eight eggs a week.

✣ Create meals **high in low-glycemic legumes**, such as lentils, chickpeas, and soybeans (try edamame, the Japanese soybeans in a pod, quickly steamed with a little salt, as a snack). These foods slow the release of sugars into the bloodstream, helping to prevent excess insulin release leading to hyperinsulinemia and its related health concerns, including poor heart health, obesity, high blood pressure, high LDL or "bad" cholesterol, and low HDL or "good" cholesterol.

- Eat a cornucopia of **fresh fruits and vegetables** teeming with phytonutrients—like carotenoids, flavonoids, and polyphenols—associated with a lower incidence of nearly all health problems, including obesity and aging.

- Eat more **slow-burning, low-glycemic vegetables**, such as asparagus, broccoli, kale, spinach, cabbage, and Brussels sprouts.

- Berries, cherries, peaches, plums, rhubarb, pears, and apples are **optimal fruits**; cantaloupes and other melons, grapes, and kiwifruit are suitable, but they contain more sugar. Organic frozen berries (brands include Cascadian Farms) can be used in protein shakes for a delicious breakfast or snack food.

- Focus on **anti-inflammatory foods**, including wild fish and other sources of omega-3 fats, red and purple berries (these are rich in polyphenols), dark green leafy vegetables, orange sweet potatoes, and nuts.

- Eat more **antioxidant-rich foods**, including orange and yellow vegetables, dark green leafy vegetables (kale, collards, spinach, etc.), anthocyanidins (berries, beets, grapes, and pomegranate), and foods containing trans-resveratrol, such as purple grapes, blueberries, bilberries, cranberries, and cherries. In fact, antioxidants are in all colorful fruits and vegetables.

- Include **detoxifying foods** in your diet, such as cruciferous vegetables (broccoli, kale, collards, Brussels sprouts, cauliflower, bok choy, Chinese cabbage, and Chinese broccoli), green tea, watercress, dandelion greens, cilantro, artichokes, garlic, citrus peels, pomegranate, and even cocoa.

- Use **herbs** such as rosemary, ginger, and turmeric, which are powerful antioxidants, anti-inflammatories, and detoxifiers.

- **Avoid excessive quantities of meat**. Use lean, organic, or grass-fed (when possible) animal products, such as eggs, beef, chicken, pork, lamb, buffalo, and ostrich. Good sources are at Whole Foods and other local health food stores. (Also see mail order options in the on-line companion guide, which you can download by going to www.ultrametabolism cookbook.com/guide.)

- **Garlic and onions** are noted for their ability to reduce cholesterol and lower blood pressure, and for their antioxidant effects. They are also anti-inflammatory and enhance detoxification.
- **A diet high in fiber** further helps to stabilize blood sugar by slowing the absorption of carbohydrates, and supports a healthy lower bowel and digestive tract. Try to gradually increase fiber to 30 to 50 grams a day and use predominantly soluble or viscous fiber (legumes, nuts, seeds, whole grains, vegetables, and fruit), which slows sugar absorption from the gut.
- **Eat a diet rich in extra-virgin olive oil**, which contains anti-inflammatory compounds and antioxidants. It should be your main oil.
- **Whole unprocessed soy products** such as soy milk, soybeans, and tofu are rich in antioxidants that can reduce cancer risk, lower cholesterol, and improve insulin and blood sugar metabolism.
- Include **nuts and seeds**, such as unsalted raw walnuts, almonds, macadamia nuts, pumpkin seeds, and flax seeds.
- And yes . . . eat **chocolate**, only the darkest, most luxurious kind, and only 2 to 3 ounces a day. It should be at least 70 percent cacao.

Decrease (or Ideally Eliminate) Your Intake of the Following Foods

- **All processed or junk foods**.
- Foods containing **refined white flour and sugar**, such as breads, cereals (including corn flakes, frosted flakes, puffed wheat, and sweetened granola), and flour-based pastas, bagels, and pastries. Occasional use of whole-grain or sprouted-grain flours can be part of a healthful diet, but should be kept to a minimum and included as part of a low-glycemic-load meal with plenty of fiber, healthy fats, and good-quality protein to minimize the effects on your blood sugar. Many who have blood sugar

problems, produce too much insulin, and tend to gain fat around the middle should enjoy products containing flour (that means any flour at all) no more than once a week.

- All foods containing **high-fructose corn syrup**.
- All **artificial sweeteners** (aspartame, sorbitol, etc.).
- **Starchy, high-glycemic cooked vegetables**, such as potatoes, corn, and root vegetables (such as rutabagas, parsnips, and turnips).
- **Processed fruit juices**, which are often loaded with sugars. (Try juicing your own carrots, celery, and beets instead, or other fruit and vegetable combinations.)
- **Processed canned vegetables** (usually very high in sodium).
- Foods containing **hydrogenated or partially hydrogenated oils** (which become trans fatty acids in the bloodstream), such as most crackers, chips, cakes, candies, cookies, doughnuts, and processed cheese.
- **Processed oils** such as corn, safflower, sunflower, peanut, and canola.
- **Red meats (unless organic or grass fed) and organ meats.** An occasional treat of red meat can be part of a healthful diet, but to attain optimal health, our diets should be predominantly plant based. The recipes with red meat included are meant to be enjoyed no more than once a week.
- **Large predatory fish and river fish**, which contain mercury and other contaminants in unacceptable amounts (including swordfish, tuna, tilefish, and shark).
- **Avoid or minimize dairy.** Substitute unsweetened, gluten-free soy milk, almond milk, or hazelnut milk beverages. While many people are intolerant of dairy, or have allergies to dairy, some can enjoy it, so I have included a few recipes with dairy. In many cases you can leave it out or substitute one of the nondairy beverages. It is especially important to use organic dairy products.
- **Limit caffeine** as much as possible (try to switch to green tea or have no more than a half cup of coffee a day).
- **Limit alcohol** to no more than three glasses of red wine per week.

Now that I have outlined the basic overall principles of UltraMetabolism, it's time for a review of each of the phases. Remember, this is an eight-week, two-phase program with a one-week preparation phase.

Preparation Phase: Let Go of Bad Habits (One Week)

We are often locked into habits without recognizing their effect on us. Most of us are drug addicts and don't realize it. Sugar, junk food, caffeine, and alcohol all affect our ability to function, and though they temporarily make us feel better, they often deplete us in a deeper way.

Taking a "drug holiday" is an important way to discover how you really feel and give yourself the opportunity to tune in to your body's signals for hunger, sleep, and relaxation. During this one-week preparation phase you eliminate sugar, high-fructose corn syrup, hydrogenated fats, junk food, alcohol, and caffeine from your diet. This alone is powerful enough to totally change your health and help you lose weight quickly. Take a risk. Even if you do nothing else, taking this step will change your life.

Phase I: Detoxify Your System (Three Weeks)

In this phase you are going to clean up your diet. Getting rid of garbage foods, moving toward a diet of whole, unprocessed foods, and eliminating foods that you may have sensitivities to will help you start the weight-loss process and reboot your metabolism.

This detoxification phase helps you quickly reset your metabolism. It is designed to further what you started in the preparation phase by removing the most common food allergens—gluten, dairy, and eggs—and introducing whole, healing foods. During the three weeks you are in this phase, you may lose six to eleven pounds and start to feel refreshed and healthier.

Besides weight loss, you can expect to feel more energy, sleep better, and get rid of chronic sinus problems, digestive problems, and headaches. Part of the healing occurs because of all the junk you are eliminating, but most occurs because you are introducing delicious, whole foods.

Phase II: Rebalance Your Metabolism and Maintain a Lifelong Healthy Metabolism (Four Weeks to Life!)

During Phase II of the program you will start to reeducate your body and program your genes to lose weight and keep it off. By doing so, you may lose an additional five to ten pounds in the first two to four weeks and then approximately a pound a week until you are at your optimal weight.

You will stick to the whole-foods diet you started in Phase I, but you will systematically reintroduce all of the foods to which you may have a hidden allergy or sensitivity. By reintroducing them this way, you can monitor their effects on your health. (If you get a stomachache or your nose stuffs up when you eat dairy, it is best to stay away from it.) This phase solidifies the hormone and immune changes in your body and allows you to reset your metabolism for the long term.

Phase II of the program is really just a four-week jumpstart for the rest of your life. Variety, fun, nourishment, pleasure, color, and wholeness are essential for making this way of eating your way of eating for life. Feel free to improvise and adapt—just stick with whole foods and you will have difficulty getting into trouble.

Although you are allowed to reintegrate all the foods you were previously avoiding in Phase II, this doesn't mean you have to stop eating the foods and recipes you loved from Phase I. You can continue to eat any Phase I recipe throughout Phase II and for the rest of your life. In fact, you will find that many of the recipes in Phase I are delicious and make you feel wonderful. Why would you want to give that up?

Because you can eat any Phase I recipe during Phase II of the program, I have "weighted" this cookbook to Phase I. That means you will find slightly more Phase I recipes than Phase II recipes overall. That way you have a lot of variety in Phase I (the more restrictive Phase of the program), and you can continue to enjoy all of these delicious recipes throughout Phase II, as well.

By the end of eight weeks (one week preparation, three weeks of the detox phase, and four weeks committed to rebalancing your metabolism for life) you may have lost 11 to 21 pounds or more, and feel so much better that you won't crave or even want to eat all the foods that you used to love but ruined your metabolism. UltraMetabolism is now yours, and you are one step closer to achieving UltraWellness.

Food Sensitivities and Well-Being

A critical part of addressing weight and health problems is dealing with food sensitivities or allergies. This is a key part of UltraMetabolism.

A large portion of our society has developed food sensitivities—reactions to foods that make us sick and cause us to gain weight. This has occurred due to many factors. It is a consequence of our nutritionally depleted diet that is full of sugar and trans fats. It is also because we eat food lacking in fiber, vitamins, minerals, and phytonutrients. Other causes include the stress we live under and the medications that we consistently overuse, such as antibiotics, antacids, and anti-inflammatories.

All these produce what is called a leaky gut (otherwise known as altered intestinal permeability). When this happens, the harmful bacteria replace the normal bacteria in our digestive system (of which there are 100 trillion), and our digestive capacity weakens. Foods are only partially digested, and the partially digested food particles "leak" through the wall of the intestinal tract.

Under that thin, one-cell-thick layer of intestinal lining is 60 percent of our immune system, ready to defend against foreign invaders such as partially digested food particles or bad bugs. Since we normally absorb foods broken down into their component parts (protein into amino acids, fats into fatty acids, and carbohydrates into simple sugars), the immune system perceives partially digested food particles that leak through your intestinal lining as foreign invaders.

Then the immune system does its job. It fights against these perceived invaders and makes us sick. In short, we have an allergic reaction to the food we eat.

But this is not a true allergy, like the hives or anaphylaxis that can come from a peanut allergy (that is called an *IgE allergy*). This is an *IgG response*. It can cause low-grade symptoms that include fatigue, resistance to weight loss, cravings and weight gain, brain fog, irritable bowel syndrome, postnasal drip, sinus congestion, allergies, headaches, eczema, psoriasis, autoimmune diseases, depression, insomnia, premenstrual syndrome, and more.

That is why the first phase of UltraMetabolism helps you eliminate the foods most likely to cause problems: gluten, dairy, and eggs. While there are tests that can help you identify these foods, and other foods to which you might react, just unloading these three common irritating foods from your diet (and thus your immune system) for a few weeks will help you see just how much they have been contributing to your suffering.

You may be thinking, "Well, I don't have one of those weird food allergies, so this isn't for me." That couldn't be further from the truth, and my 20 years' experience having astonishing success with some of the most challenging cases possible has proven this. I will simply ask you to trust me on this for a few weeks and take a leap of faith. I think you'll be amazed at how good you'll feel once these foods have been eliminated from your diet.

I also invite you to take full advantage of the one-week preparation phase of UltraMetabolism by eating only real, simple, whole foods. This means eliminating all processed, junk, and prepared foods, in addition to taking a break from stimulants like coffee and depressants like alcohol. This one week will prove to you how much impact what you eat has on your body. Your body will thank you. And I believe any doubts you have about food sensitivities being an issue for you will be eliminated as well.

After you have completed the detoxification phase of the program for three weeks, you can start adding things back to your diet slowly during Phase II and see how you feel. If you add back gluten and do fine, then great, you can keep eating it (though you may have to do so in moderation). If you add a food and feel sick, then you have the opportunity to make a choice about how you want to feel and what you eat—a choice to feel sick or to feel well based on your new knowledge of what foods you are sensitive to.

Following the program outlined in *UltraMetabolism* and eating a whole-foods diet like the one in this cookbook will go a long way toward healing a leaky gut. But sometimes it requires extra fiber, probiotics (healthy bacteria), special nutrients, and omega-3 fatty acids. Seeking out a practitioner who can help you treat a leaky gut can often help you regain your health.

The critical element for identifying food sensitivities using the elimination and reintegration techniques in *UltraMetabolism* is understanding how to transition from Phase I to Phase II of the program.

As you will see, the recipes in this book have been organized according to what phase you are on in the program. During Phase I, you can simply choose any of the recipes listed in that section, cook these delicious dishes, and enjoy them as you detoxify your system.

However, to take full advantage of the program, you will need to be careful as you transition out of Phase I and into Phase II. This is because you will want to systematically reintegrate foods.

Identifying what foods you are sensitive to is one of the single greatest gifts you can give yourself. To help you take advantage of that opportunity, let me tell you how to make this transition smooth and fluid.

Transitioning from Phase I to Phase II of UltraMetabolism

As you transition from four weeks of healing (the one-week preparation phase and the three-week detoxification phase), I encourage you to go slowly and savor the full benefits of the UltraMetabolism program.

During Phase II, your food choices will be more relaxed and more liberal. Many of the foods you eliminated during Phase I are now on the "allowed" list once more.

The temptation will be to splurge or reward yourself for your hard work by eating all the foods you love but have been avoiding. **Resist that temptation**. Overloading your system with foods that you are allergic to, or with sugar, caffeine, and alcohol, can often cause severe reactions.

Take it slowly, and choose carefully what you really want. Think about what was just a bad habit. Your body has wisdom that will awaken during your experience on Phase I of the program. Listen to this wisdom when creating your life after Phase I. Go slowly, and monitor your responses.

Remember, Phase II is going to help you rebalance your metabolism and, more important, *maintain a lifelong healthy metabolism*. If you can do this, you may start losing weight automatically and you may see health benefits you didn't expect. Going back to your old eating habits or starting to reintegrate too many foods too quickly will undermine this goal.

To help you reintroduce foods systematically as you come out of Phase I, I recommend you do the following.

What to Do When Phase I Is Over

When you've completed Phase I, you can (and should) continue many of the healthy habits you learned during this part of the program. At this point you actually have two options (one of which I did not explicitly define in *Ultra-Metabolism*).

Option 1: Continue Phase I

If you choose, you can continue the detoxification program outlined in Phase I until you achieve your ideal weight or desired health benefits.

You may continue to see major health benefits and weight loss for a full three months if you choose to continue with Phase I. After three months, you will likely have taken full advantage of this detoxification phase and you may be able to tolerate foods you are sensitive to as long as you only eat them occasionally— perhaps every three to four days.

It's usually not necessary (or even particularly advantageous) to continue with the detoxification phase for more than three months. At some point you will want to start reintegrating foods back into your diet. When you do, it's time to move on to option 2.

Option 2: End Phase I, Reintegrate Foods, and Keep Your Healthy Lifestyle

Once you are satisfied with the results you achieved during Phase I of Ultra-Metabolism, you should transition to Phase II. However, there are a number of things to keep in mind when you do.

You don't want to simply go back to your old way of eating and behaving. After all, you have suffered the consequences of that lifestyle for too long, and now you have the information you need to make healthy changes in your life.

> The single biggest gift you can give yourself at the end of this program is identifying which foods you are allergic to and which you can eat and enjoy safely.

Reintroducing foods carefully as you transition out of the program can be a very useful and educational experience. If you do it properly, you will discover which foods have been making you sick and fat. You can then keep them out of your diet and choose foods that make you thrive instead. Later, you can expand your diet to reintegrate even these items.

I will provide here a step-by-step plan for reintroducing foods into your diet. I *strongly* encourage you to follow this plan. When you end Phase I, don't give up and go back to your old lifestyle. Maintain the vital health you have worked so hard to achieve, and expand your understanding of how food works with your body by carefully reintroducing foods.

As you use the guidelines below to reintroduce foods during Phase II, keep in mind that you can continue to eat as many recipes as you wish from Phase I. It's not an "all or nothing" situation. You don't have to stop eating Phase I recipes in Phase II. I would encourage you to keep eating your favorite recipes from Phase I throughout your life. The beauty of doing so is that you don't have to worry about how *any* of those recipes might affect your health or metabolism.

Reintroduction of Potentially Allergenic Foods

When you decide to stop Phase I, whether that is after three weeks or three months, you can start reintroducing the foods you eliminated during this detox phase to see if any of them lead to symptoms or problems. This will allow you to identify problem foods and avoid them for a longer period of time, to let your immune system cool off a little more.

AN IMPORTANT WARNING

As great as you will feel at the end of Phase I, you can feel ten times worse if you suddenly go back to your old habits.

Why does this happen?

The answer is simple: Allergic reactions to the foods you eat can be *amplified* if you aren't careful.

Allergies result when a foreign protein (or antigen) joins with an antibody, causing an immune or allergic reaction. When you eliminate the foods that produce allergies, the foreign proteins or antigens suddenly drop in your blood. Then the antibodies have nothing to join on to, so you don't have an allergic reaction. This results in the feeling of wellness and health you feel at the end of Phase I.

You can get rid of the antigens quickly by stopping the problem foods. Unfortunately, the antibodies to those foods take a few months to be eliminated by the body. So when you suddenly eat that loaf of bread or hunk of cheese after you have eliminated these items from your diet during Phase I, all those antibodies floating around in your blood gang up on the foreign proteins, leading to a sudden and dramatic allergic reaction we call serum sickness.

So please follow the food reintroduction guidelines below carefully, or you can end up feeling worse than when you started. (Then again, that might be a good learning experience that will reinforce your understanding of the power food has to make you feel great or horrible.)

Keep a log of any symptoms that you experience when you reintroduce different food groups. Symptoms may occur anywhere from a few minutes to 72 hours after ingestion and can include fatigue, brain fog, mood changes, headaches, digestive upset, sleep problems, rashes, joint pains, fluid retention, and more. So pay careful attention to what is going on in your body when you reintroduce these foods.

Tracking your symptoms should guide you to which foods trigger allergic reactions in your system. When you identify the foods to which you are allergic, it's best to avoid them for 90 days. Then you can reintroduce them again, but I recommend you eat them only every four or five days, or else you could suffer from many of the symptoms they provoked once again.

Using a food log to track your symptoms and monitor your progress is an excellent way to identify which foods you can tolerate and which trigger an allergic reaction.

Note: Common symptoms may be postnasal drip; digestive problems such as bloating, gas, constipation, diarrhea, or acid reflux; headaches; joint pains; fluid retention; fatigue; brain fog; mood changes; change in sleep pattern; rashes, and more.

To help with this, I've included a food log in the downloadable companion guide, which you can access at http://www.ultrametabolismcookbook.com/guide. Or, you can use the one we've developed on our Web site at http://www.ultrawellness.com—just click on "Join" to get access to the food log as well as several other handy tools, such as a health tracker, weight tracker, and more.

Here is a plan for how to reintroduce foods over a few weeks so you can maximize the benefits of what you have just experienced.

A REMINDER AS TO WHY RECIPES ARE IN PHASE I OR PHASE II

The main foods I eliminated from Phase I are gluten, dairy, eggs, and alcohol. That is because these foods are the ones that most commonly cause allergic reactions in people. In *UltraMetabolism,* a few other foods were eliminated in Phase I, and I have followed the same approach in this cookbook. Because of their high sugar content, allergy potential, or higher saturated fat content, I have also eliminated all vinegar except rice vinegar, honey, and agave nectar, fruit juice, dried fruit, and whole chicken except chicken breasts during Phase I. For more detail on the specific foods to enjoy and avoid in Phase I and Phase II please refer to *UltraMetabolism.*

Food Reintroduction During the Four Weeks of Phase II

In *UltraMetabolism*, I explained that you could start reintegrating foods during Phase II of the program. I offered you the option of reintegrating foods in any order you chose (with the exception of dairy), to keep the process as simple as possible.

Reintegrating foods this way is absolutely healthy, and you won't suffer any adverse effects from it as long as you follow the basic guidelines mentioned above: Wait two to three days after each food you reintegrate, check for symptoms, eliminate the food for 12 weeks if you suffer from any symptoms, then reintegrate again and test for reactions.

However, there is an *even better* way to handle the reintegration process. A handful of foods are the primary culprits that cause IgG allergic reactions in people. Ideally, you will continue to stay away from these foods for the first two weeks of Phase II, and reintegrate only the foods that don't typically cause such severe reactions. Then, in the second half of Phase II, you can begin reintegrating even these foods slowly to test for reactions.

Remember, if you choose to do this, you will need to check each of the recipes outlined in this book to identify what ingredients they contain. This is very easy to do, as I have included a key at the beginning of each recipe to tell you whether or not it is gluten free, dairy free, egg free, etc. Simply refer to these notes as you choose your recipes during Phase II.

You don't *have* to do it this way; you can start reintegrating foods however you like. But if you want to take full advantage of the program and identify which foods you may be allergic to in a more systematic way, here is what I recommend you do.

Step One Reintroduction—Weeks 1 and 2

During the first two weeks of Phase II, you can begin reintegrating foods that don't typically cause severe reactions in people. That doesn't mean they won't cause reactions for you; it just means they are the safest foods to start reintegrating.

Remember to give yourself about three days to monitor reactions before you reintegrate another food. If you do have a reaction to any of these foods, stop eating the food for 90 days, after which you can experiment with reintegrating it again to see what happens.

In some cases, this will be enough to heal your leaky gut, and you may be able to eat the food again (though you may want to eat it less frequently than before so you don't run into the same problems again). In other cases, you may find certain foods continue to cause problems for you, in which case you may wish to eliminate them entirely.

Whatever you choose, by identifying foods to which you are sensitive, you rebuild a friendly relationship with food and understand the power it has to heal or harm.

Let's start with a reminder of the foods you are going to continue avoiding now and forever. Then I will tell you which foods to start reintegrating in the first two weeks of Phase II and which you should continue to avoid until weeks three and four.

Foods or Ingredients to Permanently Avoid

- ⁜ All types of refined flour products, (bagels, breads, rolls, wraps, pastas, etc.) except sprouted, whole-grain products
- ⁜ Sugar-laden foods (candy, cookies, cereals, pastries, pies, etc.)
- ⁜ High-fructose corn syrup
- ⁜ Artificial sweeteners: aspartame (Nutrasweet, Equal) saccharin (Sweet'N Low), sucralose (Splenda), and acesulfame-K (Sunette), and artificially sweetened products/beverages (cereals, diet drinks, etc.)
- ⁜ Sugar alcohols: poly-ols such as mannitol, xylitol, sorbitol, lactitol, and maltitol, etc.
- ⁜ Artificial colors
- ⁜ Hydrogenated and partially hydrogenated oils
- ⁜ Canola and peanut oils

- Fat substitutes: Olean, Olestra, Salatrim, Benefat
- Unsafe additives: potassium bromate, propyl gallate, sodium nitrite, sodium nitrate
- Caffeinated beverages: sodas, coffee, tea (except green tea), waters

Foods to Enjoy During the First Two Weeks of Phase II

- Fresh fruit (except citrus, pineapple, or dried fruit)
- More raw vegetables, like salad greens including artichokes, avocados, and olives
- Continue to enjoy organic lamb. You can also add beef (although you should keep these dense animal proteins to a minimum and consume no more than four ounces at a time).
- Grains: Continue with low-allergy grains, such as quinoa, buckwheat, and millet.
- Continue to eat vegetables, beans, and brown rice.
- Healthy oils, such as cold-pressed nut or seed oils (in addition to the extra-virgin olive oil you have been using)
- Spices: Continue to use garlic, ginger, curry or turmeric, rosemary, and fresh cilantro. You may now add any spices you enjoy.

Continue to Avoid During the First Two Weeks of Phase II

- Dairy (including milk, cheese, butter, yogurt, and sour cream)
- Gluten (including wheat, barley, rye, oats, spelt, kamut, and triticale— see www.celiac.com for a complete list of foods that include gluten)
- Eggs
- Alcohol
- Sugars in any form (including table sugar, honey, maple syrup, and corn syrup)

The foods you are going to reintegrate at this stage are the ones that most often cause problems for people. Add only one of these new foods every three to four days until you have added back all the foods you want to eat. This can take a while. Be patient. Doing this step by step will allow you to identify the problem foods for you within this list. If you experience symptoms from particular foods, you should avoid them for 90 days, then try to introduce them again.

Add Foods Back in the Following Order

- Eggs
- Gluten (barley, rye, oats, spelt, kamut, wheat—see www.celiac.com for a complete list of foods that include gluten)
- Dairy (milk, cheese, butter, yogurt)
- Alcohol (only if you enjoy it in moderation)

When you reintroduce these top food allergens, eat them at least two to three times a day for three days to see if you notice a reaction during this time (unless, of course, you notice a problem right away, in which case you should stop immediately).

As I recommended earlier, keep a log of common symptoms that occur anywhere from a few minutes to 72 hours later. If you have a reaction, note the food and eliminate it for 90 days. This will give your immune system a chance to cool off and your gut a chance to heal. In turn, this makes it more likely you will be able to tolerate more foods in the long run. However, you may find it best to eat them only occasionally (not more than once every three to four days) to keep the immune system cooled off.

After you have eliminated a food for 90 days or 12 weeks, try to it introduce again. If you still have symptoms, you may need to avoid this food long term.

Your Food Log

To help you determine which foods you have sensitivities to, I have created a food journal in which you can track your symptoms and your responses to foods.

Keeping this daily energy and food log while you are on the UltraMetabolism program is an easy and effective way to understand the relationship between the foods you eat, the way you feel, and how food affects your weight. A written record of this kind is a far more effective way to track these relationships than simply trying to remember.

This is an especially important step as you start to reintroduce foods into your diet during your transition out of Phase I of the program and into Phase II. Remember that food can affect your body and your day-to-day health in a variety of ways. The reintroduction of foods to which you may be sensitive or allergic can trigger many symptoms, including:

+ Weight gain or resistance to weight loss
+ Fluid retention
+ Nasal congestion
+ Chest congestion
+ Headaches
+ Brain fog
+ Joint aches
+ Muscle aches
+ Pain
+ Fatigue
+ Changes in skin (such as acne)
+ Changes in digestion or bowel function (such as irritable bowel syndrome)

Journaling allows you to directly see the relationship between the food you eat and the symptoms from which you suffer. Once you know this, you can change the way you eat based on your body's demands. Experiment. Fine-tune your way of eating to match your unique needs.

I encourage you to keep a food journal while you are following the four weeks of Phase II of UltraMetabolism. Remember, symptoms can be anything from physical ailments to fatigue to shifts in mood. For that reason, I suggest that you consistently record how you feel after you eat. This will give you a practical and personal understanding of how food affects you.

To help with this, I've included a food log in the downloadable companion guide, which you access at http://www.ultrametabolism cookbook.com/guide. Or, you can use the one we've developed on our Web site at http://www.ultrawellness.com—just on "Join" to get access to the food log as well as several other handy tools, including a health tracker, weight tracker, and more.

GETTING STARTED: LEARNING TO SHOP CORRECTLY AND ORGANIZE EFFECTIVELY

The recipes in this book are organized by phase to correspond to the Ultra-Metabolism program. Recipes in Phase I are designed to help you detoxify and eliminate foods to which you may have sensitivities, while those in Phase II will allow you to rebalance and maintain a healthy metabolism for life.

As you work your way through the program, pick recipes from the relevant phases so you can enjoy delicious food as you watch the effect it has on your health and weight. (Remember, you can always enjoy Phase I recipes even when you are in Phase II.) Also make sure you pay attention to the ingredients that are used in Phase II to ensure you are avoiding items to which you are sensitive.

That's all you need to do to take advantage of the delicious and healthy recipes you are about to start enjoying.

However, before you start cooking these delicious meals, I *strongly* recommend you get yourself organized and get educated about the foods in your local market.

First and foremost, you need to learn your way around the marketplace. You need to learn how to read food labels and how to determine which foods are manufactured "garbage foods" and which are whole foods that will help you heal your body and lose weight. This will allow you to take advantage of opportunities and avoid hazards in your grocery store.

Second, creating an UltraKitchen will make sticking to the program and creating delicious meals that are based on a whole-foods diet much easier. If you were climbing a mountain or planning a trek, you would make sure you had the right clothes and tools, wouldn't you? Making sure you have the right equipment for your journey to UltraWellness—lifelong health and vitality—is equally critical.

The final step is to build your UltraMetabolism Pantry so you have all the items you need for the delicious recipes in this book stocked in your kitchen. This way you can easily prepare delicious, healthful meals without having to run down to your grocery store every other day.

Getting organized, learning to navigate around your marketplace, and creating a kitchen and pantry to fit your new UltraWellness lifestyle *before* you dive into the recipes will give you the power to take full advantage of this program. It will inform your food choices and set the stage for success. Make sure to read and prepare the following *before* you dive into these delicious recipes.

Opportunities and Hazards: Navigating Stores and Labels

Reading Food Labels: If You Really Have to Buy Something Processed

While the rule "if it has a label, don't eat it" is the ideal, consumer demand has led to the creation of many clean, whole, and simple foods that actually have labels. Organic whole foods are now available in packages, cans, and boxes. They tend to be found in whole-foods stores, or the health-food section of your grocery store. (Ponder this: If there is a health-food section in the grocery store, what does that make the rest of the food sold there?) The general rule: If a food has any ingredients you don't recognize, you should likely stay away from it.

Even if it does have ingredients you are familiar with, there are times when you may want to avoid certain products in processed or manufactured foods. For example, you will want to be careful not to inadvertently include foods in your diet that aren't allowed on the UltraMetabolism program, and you will want to make sure you avoid foods you haven't officially reintegrated into your diet using the system I outlined in the previous chapter.

Be sure to read food labels carefully as you shop for the ingredients you will use in the recipes in this book. This will help you make sure you adhere to all the guidelines in the program as closely as possible. Be a smart label reader. Labels contain both the ingredients and specific (but not all) nutrition information. Here are some things of which to be aware.

Beware of marketing. Remember, the front of the label is food marketing at its cleverest. It is designed to seduce you into an emotional purchase and may contain exaggerated claims. Look for high-quality ingredients.

Where is the ingredient on the list? If the real food is at the end of the list and the sugars or salt are at the beginning, beware. The most abundant ingredient is listed first, and then the others are listed in descending order by weight.

Beware of ingredients in foods that are not labeled. Foods that are exempt from labels include foods in very small packages, foods prepared in the store, and foods made by small manufacturers.

Look for additives or problem ingredients. If a food has high-fructose corn syrup, or hydrogenated or partially hydrogenated oils, put it back on the shelf. Search for any "suspect" additives.

Look for ingredients that don't agree with you. Identify food ingredients you are sensitive to or react to, such as gluten, eggs, dairy, tree nuts, or peanuts. Be vigilant about reading labels, as these ingredients are often hidden in foods you least suspect. The labeling of common allergens is not always clear or helpful. There have been recent recommendations to improve this for consumers, as in the Food Allergen Labeling and Consumer Protection Act of 2004. (See www.celiac.com for lists of gluten-containing foods.)

Investigate unfamiliar ingredients. Use an Internet search engine or other resource to find a credible source for any unfamiliar ingredients on the label before you buy, such as carmine, quorn, or diacylglycerol. Credible Internet sources tend to be on government or educational sites ending in ".gov" or ".edu" rather than ".com."

Discover if any "functional food ingredients" are being added to the food product, such as live active cultures, beta-glucan (a viscous fiber), or plant sterols. Though they may be helpful, more often than not they are "window dressing," present in small amounts, and with minimal value, except to the marketing department of the manufacturer. Examples of this include live active cultures added to high-sugar, high-fat yogurts or vitamins, "vitamin enriched" sugar-laden cereals, and ginkgo in potato chips. In other words, it's best to get healthful, functional food ingredients from their whole-food sources, rather than as additives to otherwise nutritionally deficient foods.

Would your great-grandmother have served this food? Finally, before you analyze the numbers, ask yourself if this food could have been served at your great-grandmother's table. She served only real food.

Understanding the Nutrition Label: Think Low GL and High PI

Glycemic load, or GL, is a measure of how quickly a food enters your bloodstream. Low GL leads to better health. Phytonutrient index, or PI, refers to the amount of colorful plant pigments and compounds in a food that help prevent disease and promote health. High PI leads to better health.

Look at the serving size and determine if this is your "typical" portion, as labels can be deceiving. For example, a cereal may state "¾ cup serving," when your typical portion is 1½ cups. Or worse, it may say "2 servings," when typically people consume the whole amount in the container or bottle. Have you ever known four people to share one pint of Häagen Daz ice cream?

Are the calories high GL or low GL? The total amount of carbohydrates is less important than where they come from. If they are found in foods with a low GL and high PI, they will have a very different effect on your appetite and weight than foods that are quickly absorbed and have few nutrients and fiber.

Start with fiber. It is one of the main factors that determine the all-important glycemic load, and it can also give you a clue about the phytonutrient index. Many packaged foods have no fiber. If convenience items such as soups, entrées, or snacks are missing this key fiber factor, leave them on the shelf.

Look at total carbohydrates. Remember that it's the type of carbs that matters most. If they are from whole, plant foods that contain plenty of fiber or have a low GL, their effect is very different from that of fiberless foods. The same amount of carbohydrates from a can of beans or from a can of Coke affects the body in very different ways.

Where are the good fats? Monounsaturated and omega-3 polyunsaturated fats should dominate this category, with minimal amounts of saturated fat and zero trans fats (present on food labels from 2006 on).

Beware that small amounts of trans fat are STILL permitted in packaged foods as long as the food contains less than 0.5 grams per serving. But if you eat that food frequently, or eat more than one serving (which is usually the case), you may get a load of trans fats. Therefore, look carefully at the label even if it says "zero trans fats." Look for the words *hydrogenated* or *partially hydrogenated*. If you see those words, put the item back on the shelf.

Unfortunately, the omega-3 fats are rarely listed on the label. They are part of the polyunsaturated fat family, but they come from the good side of the family (they are anti-inflammatory; bad poly-unsaturated or omega-6 fats are inflammatory. Other processed and refined oils that are less than healthful also show up in this section of the label, including corn oil and safflower oil.)

Now for the "Nutrition Facts" on the label:

Cholesterol. Your liver makes more cholesterol in an hour than you ever eat in a day. More cholesterol is produced in the body from eating sugar than from eating fat. There is little correlation between dietary cholesterol and blood cholesterol, and little reason to worry about this number on food labels. Yes, a surprising fact perhaps to many of you, but true.

Protein. If you eat a variety of whole foods you won't have to worry about protein, because whole foods such as beans, soy foods, nuts, seeds, whole grains, and lean animal foods contain plenty of protein.

Sodium. If you are sodium sensitive, use this simple guideline: Double the calories to get an accurate estimate of how much sodium should be in the serving (for example, 150 calories per serving, maximum sodium per serving 300 milligrams). There's an exception to this rule: very low-calorie foods, such as some vegetables without added salt. Many processed foods have far more sodium than this.

You will need to prepare fresh foods at home to recondition your palate to whole foods naturally low in sodium. The recommended daily intake for the average person is 1500 milligrams, or less than the amount in one teaspoon of salt (2400 mg). That includes salt added at the table, in cooking at the factory, or in a fast-food kitchen (which is where most of our salt intake comes from—hidden in the processed and fast foods we consume, such as packaged meats, canned soup, and even cottage cheese!).

We should consume about ten times the amount of potassium, mostly from plant foods (such as bananas, potatoes, spinach, and almonds), as sodium in our diet, yet we do just the inverse. We eat ten times as much salt or sodium as potassium from table salt, processed foods, and restaurant foods.

Calcium. Add a zero to the calcium percentage on the label. This equals the milligrams of calcium per serving, because the "% Daily Value" for calcium is based on 1000 milligrams. For example: 2 percent equals 20 milligrams calcium, and 30 percent equals 300 milligrams. Remember that calcium is the only nutrient to which this rule pertains.

Other nutrients. B-12, iron, zinc, and other nutrients may have been added to the food product to enhance nutrient levels and will be listed on the label if the product was "fortified." Many junk foods have vitamins or nutrients added. Beware: they can make you feel fine about eating bad-quality foods, yet they have no real benefit.

What Are Organic Foods, Whole Foods, and Whole Grains?

Part of the power of the UltraMetabolism program is that it takes you a step toward the evolutionary roots of the human diet. People evolved eating whole, organic foods. Our bodies are designed to properly digest these kinds of foods, not the highly processed "garbage foods" on the market today.

Unfortunately, our culture is so far from this fundamental understanding of how to eat that you may not be completely clear on what I mean by "whole, organic foods." This problem is complicated by the fact that in the world of organic food, a lot of different terminology has sprung up that describes the degree to which the food has been processed.

To help clarify the definitions in the book as well as the ones you will see on your supermarket shelf, I have compiled the information that follows. Take it with you when you buy groceries until you feel comfortable with all the terminology that is currently used.

Whole foods are foods as they are found in nature—fresh, unprocessed, and simple. They are foods that come from a farmer's field, not a food chemist's laboratory. These include the following:

High-fiber Foods

- Beans
- Whole grains
- Vegetables
- Fruits
- Nuts
- Seeds

Quality Proteins

- Beans, including whole soy foods such as tofu, edamame, and tempeh
- Nuts
- Eggs
- Fish
- Lean poultry, lamb, pork, or beef (preferably organic, grass-fed, or range-fed)

Healthy Fats

- Fish oil
- Extra-virgin olive oil and olives
- Avocados
- Coconut oil (organic extra-virgin)
- Healthy oils: walnut, avocado, grapeseed, and flax oil
- Nuts and seeds, and nut and seed butters

Healthy Carbohydrates

- Vegetables
- Fruits
- Beans
- Whole grains

What Is Organic?

There are a number of terms related to "organic" food products. The following information should help you understand what these terms mean and assist you in choosing quality food products that are raised naturally and have minimal exposure to pesticides, herbicides, or antibiotics.

Organic: Organic foods are agricultural products that have been grown and treated in a way that is in closer harmony with the natural ecology of the area in which they are grown. Organic produce is grown with few pesticides, in a way that keeps the soil fertile and the water clean.

Certified Organic: Foods that are certified organic have been held to very strict standards by the National Organics Standards Board. These standards include a restriction on the use of chemicals of any kind.

Free-Range: This refers to a way of raising feed animals (chickens, pigs, and cattle) in which the animal is not confined to a feedlot, stockyard, coop, or barn. Animals raised in confined conditions tend to have more diseases, are less healthy, and are fed an unnatural diet. Thus, they are full of poor-quality saturated fats. Free-range animals, while not necessarily completely free of antibiotics (used to keep disease down where large groups of animals are present), tend to be healthier.

Grass-Fed Beef or Meat: This beef comes from cattle that spend their lives roaming and eating grass in a pasture. Grass-fed cattle are not closed up in a stockyard, which means they have much less need for antibiotics. They move more and eat a healthier, more natural diet, which means they are leaner. When you eat grass-fed beef, you are eating leaner meat that has fewer saturated fats than feedlot cattle.

Grass-Finished Beef or Meat: Not all grass-fed cattle have been grass-fed their entire lives. In some cases, marketers pass off cattle that have spent part of their lives in a feedlot as "grass-fed." These cows may have eaten some grass, or spent some time in a pasture, but they have also been kept in feedlots. "Grass-finished" cattle have never seen a feedlot. They spend their entire lives in a pasture. This means they are the cleanest form of beef you can find.

What Is a Grain?

Whole grain: A whole grain is the "fruit" of grasses that used to be wild, such as oats, wheat, rye, barley, and rice. Eating a refined grain is like eating a piece of fruit without the skin or seeds—often two of the most nutritious parts. Each whole grain has a bran (skin), an endosperm (the inside of the fruit), and a germ (the seed). The endosperm is where all the starch (sugar) is, the bran is the source of the fiber, and the germ is the source of vitamins and minerals. When choosing whole grains, look for brown rice, steel-cut oats, rye, barley, buckwheat, amaranth, or quinoa.

Sprouted grain: A sprouted grain is a whole grain soaked in water, which starts the germination process and makes the grain easier to digest. It is more slowly broken down in the gut and has a lower glycemic load than refined flour or grains. Try sprouted-grain bread or tortillas.

Refined grain: A grain that has the bran and germ removed is pure starch and is quickly absorbed, leading to surges in blood sugar and swings in appetite. It is commonly known as white rice, white flour, wheat flour or white bread, or oat-meal. Don't eat this!

Creating Your Own UltraKitchen

If you were climbing a mountain or planning a trek into unknown territory, you would make sure you had the right clothing and tools. You would study the map before you set out. The journey of self-discovery, the journey that will take you to a healthy metabolism, requires some preparation and equipment. Some special tools and instructions will make your journey successful.

Let's start with your kitchen. Getting the basic equipment makes food preparation easier and faster, as will learning what to clean from your pantry and what hazards to avoid in the marketplace. The suggestions and guidelines offered here will provide practical tools for your adventure into a healthy metabolism—an UltraMetabolism.

Arm Yourself With the Proper Tools

Consider this equipment a toolkit for taking care of your body. You can substitute or make do with other tools if need be, but I would strongly recommend that you consider purchasing the following items if you don't already have them.

I would also recommend that you buy the best-quality tools possible as you build your kitchen. If you were climbing a mountain, you would buy boots that would last for the duration. The items in this list are as vital to your health as an excellent pair of boots would be if you were to go mountain climbing. These tools can last you a lifetime if you start with quality items and take proper care of them.

I consider the following to be the basic essential hardware for the care and feeding of a human being (or at least the feeding!).

- A set of good-quality knives
- Wooden cutting boards—one for animal products, another for fruits and vegetables
- An 8-inch nonstick sauté pan
- A 12-inch nonstick sauté pan (Nonstick pans can vary in quality. Buy the highest quality, such as Calphalon or All-Clad, because of the health risks of poorer-quality nonstick pans using Teflon.)
- An 8-quart stockpot
- A 2-quart saucepan with lid
- A 4-quart saucepan with lid
- An 11-inch-square nonstick (non-Teflon) stovetop griddle
- Dutch oven
- Grill pan
- 3 or 4 cookie or baking sheets
- A food processor
- A blender
- An immersion blender
- An instant-read chef's thermometer
- A can opener
- A coffee grinder for flaxseed
- Wire whisks
- Spring tongs
- A fish spatula
- Rubber spatulas
- Natural parchment paper

The UltraMetabolism Cookbook

- Assorted measuring cups (1 quart, 1 pint, and 1 cup), dry and liquid style
- A lemon/citrus reamer
- A food mill/potato ricer
- Microplanes in assorted sizes

Rid Your Kitchen of Fat-Burning Enemies

Before you purchase the items you need to start the program, take an afternoon to cleanse your cabinets of the items that are harmful to your health and metabolism. This includes eliminating toxic fats and sugars from your cabinets so that you won't "accidentally" add them to a recipe.

Start by throwing into the trash all items containing hydrogenated and partially hydrogenated fats and high-fructose corn syrup. Those two changes alone can radically alter your life by changing your cells and your metabolism. Reading the labels (see the section above) on each of the food products in your cabinets and refrigerator will tell you which ones contain these ingredients.

Tips and Tricks

Over the years, working with the best nutritionist in the country, Kathie Swift, I have accumulated some tips and tricks to eat well and feel well. I offer them to you here.

Learn the Best Brands

By eliminating what you don't need anymore, you will open up space in your refrigerator and cabinets for healthier alternatives. If you carefully read the labels of the foods you buy, in time you will develop a sense for which products contain real, whole foods and which don't.

Local food co-ops or national chains such as Whole Foods, Trader Joe's, and Wild Oats have many excellent products that fit into the UltraMetabolism program and the recipes in this book. Be proactive and urge your supermarket chain to carry these types of products. Buy foods that have not been or are only minimally processed. I recommend choosing organic foods whenever possible to reduce exposure to pesticides and increase your intake of vitamin, minerals, antioxidants, and phytonutrients.

Choose Organic, Hormone- and Antibiotic-Free Food

Buy antibiotic- and hormone-free animal products, such as dairy products, poultry, and red meat, whenever possible. Avoid eating fish that contain high levels of mercury, such as swordfish, tilefish, shark, king mackerel, and fresh tuna (canned tuna, especially chunk light, is lower in mercury). I recommend you eat fish with the least mercury, including blue crab (mid-Atlantic), flounder, sole, wild salmon, sardines, herring, anchovies, and shrimp. Check periodic updates on seafood safety on www.ewg.org and www.oceansalive.com.

Buy a variety of seasonally fresh, locally grown, and, whenever possible, certified organic produce. Though organic food is generally more expensive, the benefits are worth it. Organic food does not contain the high levels of pesticides, hormones, and antibiotics found in conventional foods. Research indicates that organic foods also have more nutrients than foods grown conventionally.

The following is a priority list for purchasing organic produce based on data from the Environmental Working Group (www.ewg.org):

- Apples
- Apricots
- Cantaloupe
- Celery
- Cherries
- Corn
- Cucumbers
- Grapes
- Peaches
- Pears
- Red and green peppers
- Spinach
- Strawberries

Some nonorganically grown items in your local grocery store are still relatively healthy to eat. If you can't completely stick to organically grown produce (either because your grocery store doesn't carry it or because the cost is prohibitive), the following eleven items are generally considered the products that are least contaminated by pesticides. While I encourage you to buy as much organic produce as you can, if you can't, these are items you would probably be safe purchasing in a conventionally grown form.

- Asparagus
- Avocados
- Bananas
- Broccoli
- Cauliflower
- Kiwis
- Mangos
- Onions
- Papayas
- Pineapples
- Peas (sweet)

Check out the Environmental Working Group Web site (www.ewg.org) for further updates. You can also reduce your exposure to pesticides and bacteria by washing your produce well. Prepare a vegetable wash solution by adding one teaspoon of mild soap or one tablespoon of cider vinegar to one gallon of water. Wash your vegetables in this solution and rinse well. Use a vegetable brush on potatoes, sweet potatoes, carrots, or other hard produce whose skin you plan to eat.

Seek Out These Antioxidant Powerhouses

Scientists continue to learn more about measuring antioxidants in foods, referred to as ORAC (oxygen radical absorbance capacity), or the ability of the food to soak up damaging free radical molecules (in a test tube). Be aware that with ongoing research, ORAC values may change and new foods may be added or change place on the list.

In the meantime, have fun with this Top 20 list of antioxidant foods. Be sure to include plenty of these on your shopping lists. How many of these foods do you like? Were there any that surprised you by making the Top 20, such as russet potatoes, which have been maligned by many popular diet books? Which ones might you now be more likely to introduce?

1. Small red beans (dried legumes)
2. Wild blueberries
3. Red kidney beans

4. Pinto beans
5. Cultivated blueberries
6. Cranberries
7. Cooked artichokes
8. Blackberries
9. Prunes
10. Raspberries
11. Strawberries
12. Red Delicious apples
13. Granny Smith apples
14. Pecans
15. Sweet cherries
16. Black plums
17. Cooked russet potatoes
18. Black beans
19. Plums
20. Gala apples

DRINK CLEAN WATER

Contact your local water department to find out about the quality of your drinking water. Consider a water-purifying system such as a reverse osmosis filter for your home. If you drink bottled water, choose glass or clear, hard, durable plastic containers (versus soft, opaque, thin, easily bendable plastic). Soft plastics tend to release toxic chemicals, including phythalates and bisphenol A, which have been linked to hormonal disorders and infertility.

AVOID food products that contain:

- Hydrogenated or partially hydrogenated oils
- High-fructose corn syrup
- Artificial sweeteners such as aspartame, saccharin or acesulfame-K, cyclamate, neotame, and saccharin sucralose
- Sugar alcohols such as sorbitol, mannitol, xylitol, and maltitol, which often cause gas and intestinal upset
- Artificial fats such as olestra
- Artificial colorings (dyes, such as FD & C Yellow No. 5 and Red No. 3)
- Preservatives such as BHA and BHT
- Brominated vegetable oil (BVO), a known toxic additive that is found in some citrus sodas
- Heptyl paraben, a preservative used in beer and some noncarbonated drinks
- Hydrogenated starch hydrolysate (a sweetener)
- Hydrolyzed vegetable protein, a flavor enhancer added to instant soups, sauce mixes, and hot dogs
- Monosodium glutamate, a flavor enhancer added to many foods that has been shown to cause adverse reactions in some people, perhaps by over-stimulating brain activity
- Propyl gallate, a preservative found in edible fats, such as mayonnaise, oils, shortening, baked goods, and dried meats
- Potassium bromate, a flavor enhancer found in breads and banned in several countries as a carcinogen
- Sodium nitrite and sodium nitrate, preservatives that have been linked to cancer, found in processed meats
- Sulfites (sulfur dioxide and sodium bisulfite), preservatives found in wine, dried fruit, instant potatoes, French fries, pizza, and other foods, linked to headaches and severe allergic reactions in some

Check out the Center for Science in the Public Interest's Web site for further information and updates: www.cspinet.org (click on Chemical Cuisine).

Avoid These Foods

You can eat these foods from time to time (once or twice a week), but make sure you are not eating them too often.

- Refined flour products ("wheat flour" or "enriched wheat flour" is essentially the same as white flour, unless the label explicitly lists "whole wheat flour" as the first ingredient). Small amounts of whole sprouted-grain products are fine occasionally.
- Refined sugars. Refined sugar is most often described as sugar separated from the stalk of sugarcane, or from the beet root of the sugar beet. The sugar-containing juice is extracted, processed, and dried into sugar crystals.
- Highly saturated animal fat in meats (fatty meats, deli meats, sausage, etc.) and dairy fat.
- Alcohol in moderation (should be avoided altogether by alcohol-sensitive individuals).

Suggestions for Success

When you are preparing and cooking your meals, keep these suggestions in mind. They can make cooking a relaxing and enjoyable experience, allowing food to become your ally instead of your enemy and your kitchen to become a sanctuary instead of a battleground.

- With a little patience and practice, you will feel very comfortable in the kitchen.
- Get organized, think through your week ahead, and take one day each week to spend a few hours shopping and cooking.
- Carefully create a shopping list before you head to the store.

- When you come home from the store, organize your groceries in the refrigerator and pantry.
- Don't be intimidated by the recipes; simply read over each recipe carefully before starting to cook.
- Put on some fun music, and wash and chop vegetables on the weekend or the day before and store in zip-top bags in the refrigerator. You are much more likely to eat them if they are all ready to cook.
- Multitask while in the kitchen. Simmer some soup or cook a grain for the next day while preparing dinner.
- Also, double or even triple the recipes and freeze some for later use. Having a meal ready to go in the freezer is as good as money in the bank!

Putting It Together to Build the Perfect Kitchen

Remember that your kitchen is one of the most important rooms in your home. It is the place where you prepare the food that is going to nourish and sustain you and your family. When your kitchen is out of balance or you don't have the right tools, it is difficult to prepare healthy meals that turn on the genes that keep you healthy and help you lose weight.

As you start on the UltraMetabolism program, try to implement some (if not all) of the tips in this section so your kitchen and the time that you spend preparing food can be enjoyable and rewarding. Getting re-enchanted with nourishing, delicious food, with the pleasure of eating, is so important—it is at the center of human life and belongs in an UltraKitchen, not the front seat of your minivan!

Building Your UltraMetabolism Pantry

Eating the UltraMetabolism way does not require anything that cannot be found in your local market. Below are suggestions of the types of ingredients that I prefer for reasons of both health and flavor. Always choose whole, fresh foods and, whenever possible, buy local, seasonal fruits and vegetables that are organically grown.

Buy seasonally fresh, locally grown, and organic produce whenever possible, as well as antibiotic- and hormone-free organic poultry, dairy products, and red meat. Buy as many organic foods as your budget will allow. (Research indicates that organic foods have more nutrients and do not have the high levels of pesticides, hormones, and antibiotics of conventional foods.)

Organic fruits and vegetables are also available frozen and canned. I used organic canned beans and tahini, fresh organic produce, organic poultry; grass-fed meat; organic frozen fruits and vegetables and organic dairy products in the testing and development of these recipes. If you can't buy all organic products, see the list of products above in the section on building an UltraKitchen for organic priorities.

For information about buying organic produce, check the Environmental Working Group's Web site at www.ewg.org, and for information on seafood safety, check www.ewg.org or www.oceansalive.org.

Fish and Seafood

Wild, not farmed, seafood is preferred.

Poultry

Poultry raised without hormones or antibiotics is recommended. Remove the skin from poultry before cooking.

Ground Poultry Products

Make sure to use only high-quality, organic ground poultry products.

Meat

Buy as much grass-fed or grass-finished, organic, hormone-free meat as your budget will allow. Trim all visible fat from the meat before cooking. Remember, red meat should be enjoyed no more than once a week in Phase II.

Eggs

Organic omega-3 enriched eggs are a "functional food" readily available at your local supermarket. They come from chickens fed a diet rich in algae or flaxseed as the original source of these healthy fats. In this instance, the eggs are "what the chicken ate." The egg yolks are rich in omega-3 fatty acids. Egg yolks, once shunned for their cholesterol content, are rich in many nutrients including choline, a phospholipid that is a key component of cells and is important for a healthy nervous system.

Eggs are to be used only in Phase II, and only after you have properly reintroduced them into your diet so you can test for food sensitivities.

Water

Contact your local water department to find out about the quality of your drinking water.

For cooking and drinking, I suggest you use filtered water in all recipes. Consider a water-purifying system such as a reverse osmosis filter for your home. (The resources list in the downloadable *UltraMetabolism Cookbook Companion Guide* includes these and other important items that will improve your UltraKitchen even further. You can access the guide at http://www.ultrametabolismcookbook /guide.) If you drink bottled water, choose glass or clear, hard durable plastic containers (versus soft, opaque, thin, easily bendable plastic.) Soft plastics release toxic chemicals called phlalates.

Condiments

Mayonnaise
You can use organic soy mayonnaise in the recipes in this book, or you may prefer to make your own mayonnaise (see the recipe on page 258). Traditional egg-based mayonnaise can be used only in Phase II recipes but should not be used in Phase I of the program. Soy mayo can be used in both, but make sure you check

the label to see what's in it. Even in Phase II, remember to read the label of any mayonnaise you choose to buy.

Soy sauce (Tamari)
I recommend low-sodium, wheat-free or gluten-free tamari.

Miso
Several recipes in this cookbook call for miso. This is a Japanese condiment that is often used to make soups and is also used as flavoring for many different recipes. It can be found in the Japanese or Asian section of many different markets.

When buying miso make sure you choose a gluten-free version. These are usually made from chickpeas or brown rice. Read the labels to make sure you know what you are getting.

Red chili paste
I used a gluten-free red chili paste called Thai Kitchen Red Chili Paste that is free of sulfites and other preservatives. Other brands may work as well. Make sure you read the labels to find a version of this sauce that is "clean."

Tahini
Tahini is a paste made from ground sesame seeds; it is an ingredient in hummus and has wonderful flavor.

Seasonings

Kosher salt
Use kosher salt for all your salt needs.

Fresh herbs
For best results, use the freshest of herbs. Some herbs, such as basil, are added at the end of the cooking process for maximum flavor. Most herbs are high in antioxidants and transform the flavor of many foods.

Broth or stock

Most recipes can be made successfully with either broth or stock. Buy organic reduced- or low-sodium broth or stock. Also check to make sure the brand you choose is gluten-free. If you make your own, use salt sparingly. You can adjust the seasonings for flavor later during the cooking process.

Canned or boxed foods

Occasionally I recommend canned beans, tomatoes, or tomato juice for convenience. I recommend using organic low- or no-sodium versions to reduce your overall salt intake. See resources for specific brands.

Fresh lemon and lime juice

Use fresh lemons and limes. A citrus reamer is excellent for extracting the juice. Strain the seeds from the juice.

Agave nectar

Agave nectar, sometimes sold as agave syrup, is a light-colored syrup with a neutral flavor. It is used in recipes as a sweetener during Phase II.

Pomegranate molasses

This is a form of molasses containing additional benefits that come from the pomegranates from which it is made. You also get to enjoy the wonderful flavor of this health-promoting fruit.

Dark chocolate

Choose a dark chocolate, with a minimum 70 percent cacao content.

Oils

Olive oil

Use extra-virgin olive oil. Buy the best extra-virgin oil your budget allows.

Sesame oil

Recipes specify either light or dark sesame oil.

It's now time to start becoming friends with food again and use it as an ally on your journey to UltraWellness. The recipes that follow are your key to doing that. Choose recipes based on the phase you are in. Then enjoy these delicious foods as you journey to the thin, fit, healthy you that's waiting to emerge.

The

Recipes

Guacamole

Phase I: Detox
Gluten Free
Dairy Free
Quick
Vegetarian
Egg Free

Serves 10
Serving size: ¼ cup
Yield: 2½ cups
Prep time: 20 minutes
Cook time: none

This is everyone's favorite. If you prefer more heat, just add more minced jalapeño pepper. It's tasty with sliced fresh, raw vegetables or as an accompaniment to plain grilled chicken or fish.

2 large avocados (about 9 ounces each), peeled, pitted, and cut into ¾-inch pieces

½ cup diced red onion

2 medium tomatoes, chopped

5 tablespoons chopped cilantro

1 teaspoon minced jalapeño pepper

1 teaspoon fresh lime juice

½ teaspoon kosher salt

Place all ingredients in a medium bowl. Gently mix until blended, but still chunky. Serve with desired accompaniments.

Nutritional Analysis

Per ¼-cup serving: 68 Calories, 5 g Fat, 0.7 g Sat, 0 mg Chol, 3 g Fiber, 1 g Protein, 5 g Carb, 144 mg Sodium

Hummus

Phase I: Detox
Gluten Free
Dairy Free
Quick
Vegetarian
Egg Free

Serves 10
Serving size: ¼ cup
Yield: 2½ cups
Prep time: 20 minutes
Cook time: none

This dip is garlicky, lemony, and even better drizzled with the optional extra-virgin olive oil. Pair with sliced raw vegetables for a nice appetizer, or serve as part of an appetizer buffet.

1 (15-ounce) can chickpeas or 2 cups cooked chickpeas

½ cup tahini

5 tablespoons extra-virgin olive oil

¼ cup fresh lemon juice

4 medium cloves garlic

½ teaspoon kosher salt

¼ teaspoon freshly ground black pepper

⅛ teaspoon ground red pepper

1 tablespoon extra-virgin olive oil (optional)

Drain and rinse the chickpeas, reserving ½ cup of the liquid from the can or from the cooking process.

Combine the chickpeas, tahini, extra-virgin olive oil, lemon juice, garlic, salt, and black and red pepper in the bowl of a food processor fitted with a metal blade. Process until the mixture is smooth. If the mixture is too thick, add 1 to 2 tablespoons of the reserved liquid for desired consistency. Remove to a serving dish, and drizzle with 1 tablespoon extra-virgin olive oil before serving, if desired.

Nutritional Analysis

Per ¼-cup serving: 213 Calories, 17 g Fat, 2.2 g Sat, 0 mg Chol,

4 g Fiber, 5 g Protein, 12 g Carb, 213 mg Sodium

Indian Spiced Cashews

These have a subtle curry flavor. They are best served warm on the day they're made.

2 cups raw, unsalted cashews

2 teaspoons extra-virgin olive oil

1 teaspoon Madras curry powder

½ teaspoon kosher salt

½ teaspoon ground coriander

½ teaspoon ground cumin

½ teaspoon ground cinnamon

½ teaspoon ground fenugreek

½ teaspoon ground chile pepper

Phase I: Detox
Gluten Free
Dairy Free
Quick
Vegetarian
Egg Free

Serves 8
Serving size: ¼ cup
Yield: 2 cups
Prep time: 10 minutes
Cook time: 10 minutes

Preheat the oven to 300 degrees F.

Toss the cashews and extra-virgin olive oil together on a baking sheet.

In a small bowl, mix together the curry powder, salt, coriander, cumin, cinnamon, fenugreek, and ground chile pepper. Sprinkle over the cashews, turning the cashews to coat thoroughly.

Bake for about 10 minutes, until golden brown and fragrant. Serve warm.

Nutritional Analysis

Per ¼-cup serving: 210 Calories, 17 g Fat, 3.3 g Sat, 0 mg Chol,

1 g Fiber, 5 g Protein, 12 g Carb, 123 mg Sodium

Marinated Olives Provençal

Phase I: Detox
Gluten Free
Dairy Free
Vegetarian
Egg Free

Serves 8
Serving size: 2 tablespoons
Yield: 1 cup olives
Prep time: 10 minutes,
plus several hours
marinating time
Cook time: none

These olives are herbaceous and somewhat spicy. Try a mix of large black and green olives such as Kalamata, Gaeta, or Cerignola.

1 cup mixed olives

¼ cup extra-virgin olive oil

2 strips of orange zest, each 1½ inches long

2 medium cloves garlic, crushed with a knife

1 teaspoon fresh lemon juice

¾ teaspoon crushed red pepper flakes

¼ teaspoon freshly ground black pepper

2 sprigs of thyme

In a medium bowl, mix together all ingredients and refrigerate for several hours, or overnight.

Bring to room temperature, and remove the garlic cloves before serving.

Nutritional Analysis

Per 2-tablespoon serving: 104 Calories, 10.5 g Fat, 1.4 g Sat, 0 mg Chol,

0.8 g Fiber, 0.2 g Protein, 1.5 g Carb, 231 mg Sodium

Roasted Red Pepper Dip

The smoky flavor of the roasted peppers is enhanced by the addition of garlic, herbs, and sun-dried tomatoes. For more fiber, serve with fresh, raw vegetables, especially pieces of fresh fennel, or put a tablespoon or two on grilled fish or chicken to make a delicious sauce.

Phase I: Detox
Gluten Free
Dairy Free
Quick
Vegetarian
Egg Free

Serves 8
Serving size: 2 tablespoons
Yield: 1 cup
Prep time: 15 minutes
Cook time: none

¼ cup chopped basil (about 10 large leaves)

¼ cup chopped parsley

1 medium clove garlic

1 cup roasted red peppers (about 8 ounces) (page 150)

½ cup chopped brine-cured black olives, such as Kalamata or Gaeta

¼ cup extra-virgin olive oil

2 oil-packed sun-dried tomatoes, drained

2 teaspoons fresh lemon juice

¼ teaspoon kosher salt

½ teaspoon freshly ground black pepper

Pinch of crushed red pepper flakes

Combine the basil, parsley, and garlic in the bowl of a food processor fitted with a metal blade. Process until finely chopped. Add the red peppers, olives, extra-virgin olive oil, sun-dried tomatoes, lemon juice, salt, pepper, and red pepper flakes. Process until smooth.

Nutritional Analysis

Per 2-tablespoon serving: 86 Calories, 8 g Fat, 1.2 g Sat, 0 mg Chol,

1 g Fiber, 1 g Protein, 3 g Carb, 140 mg Sodium

Roasted Tomato and Garlic Spread

This earthy, flavorful spread can be served as an appetizer with raw vegetables.

Phase I: Detox
Gluten Free
Dairy Free
Vegetarian
Egg Free

Serves 4
Serving size: ¼ cup
Yield: 1 cup
Prep time: 15 minutes
Cook time: 30 minutes

½ medium-size head of garlic
¼ cup plus ½ teaspoon extra-virgin olive oil
¼ teaspoon kosher salt
½ teaspoon freshly ground black pepper
1 pound grape or cherry tomatoes, cut into quarters, or halves if very small
2 teaspoons minced flat-leaf parsley
4 fresh basil leaves, cut into thin strips (about 2 teaspoons)

Preheat the oven to 400 degrees F.

Cut the head of garlic in half horizontally. Place the garlic on a piece of aluminum foil. Drizzle with ½ teaspoon extra-virgin olive oil and sprinkle with a pinch of salt and pepper. Wrap the garlic tightly in the foil and place on a large baking sheet.

In a medium bowl, stir together the tomatoes, ¼ cup extra-virgin olive oil, the salt, and pepper. Spread the tomato mixture in a single layer on the baking sheet with the wrapped garlic. Place in the oven and roast for about 30 minutes, until the tomatoes start to brown.

Remove the tomatoes from the baking sheet and place them in a small bowl. Remove the garlic from the foil. Squeeze the individual garlic cloves from their skins and add to the tomatoes. Stir in the parsley and basil.

Nutritional Analysis

Per ¼-cup serving: 165 Calories, 14 g Fat, 2 g Sat, 0 mg Chol, 2 g Fiber, 2 g Protein, 9 g Carb, 128 mg Sodium

Rosemary White Bean Dip with Red Pepper and Fennel Strips

This appetizer is simple to prepare. Drizzle extra-virgin olive oil on top for even better flavor. The red pepper strips and fennel make a flavorful and colorful accompaniment to the dip.

1 (15-ounce) can Great Northern beans, drained and rinsed

5 tablespoons extra-virgin olive oil

2 teaspoons minced garlic (about 2 medium cloves)

1 teaspoon chopped rosemary

¼ teaspoon kosher salt

¾ teaspoon coarsely ground black pepper

2 medium red bell peppers, cored, seeded, and cut into strips

1 bulb fennel, cored and cut into strips

Phase I: Detox
Gluten Free
Dairy Free
Quick
Vegetarian
Egg Free

Serves 5
Serving size: ¼ cup
Yield: 1¼ cups
Prep time: 25 minutes
Cook time: none

Combine the beans, extra-virgin olive oil, garlic, rosemary, salt, and pepper in the bowl of a food processor fitted with a metal blade. Process until smooth, scraping the sides of the bowl if necessary.

Drizzle with additional extra-virgin olive oil before serving with the sliced red pepper and fennel.

Nutritional Analysis

Per ¼-cup serving: 202 Calories, 14g Fat, 2.0 g Sat, 0 mg Chol,

6 g Fiber, 5 g Protein, 18 g Carb, 450 mg Sodium

Super Bowl Sunday Dip

Phase I: Detox
Gluten Free
Dairy Free
Quick
Vegetarian
Egg Free

Serves 12
Serving size: ¼-cup portion
Yield: 3 cups
Prep time: 20 minutes
Cook time: none

A remake of the classic seven-layer dip, this is a super dairy- and gluten-free party food. Serve with sliced fresh vegetables.

1 cup vegetarian refried beans

1 medium avocado, chopped (about ¾ cup)

3 tablespoons minced red onion

2 teaspoons fresh lime juice

1 teaspoon finely chopped oregano

1 teaspoon minced jalapeño pepper

¼ cup minced cilantro

½ teaspoon kosher salt

½ cup diced roasted red bell pepper (page 150)

½ cup chopped tomatoes

Spread the refried beans in a shallow bowl or platter.

In a small bowl, stir together the avocado, red onion, lime juice, oregano, jalapeño, 2 tablespoons of the cilantro, and the salt. Spread the mixture on the refried beans.

Sprinkle the roasted red pepper over the avocado mixture and top with the tomatoes and remaining cilantro.

Nutritional Analysis

Per ¼-cup serving: 45 Calories, 3 g Fat, 0.5 g Sat, 0 mg Chol, 2 g Fiber, 1 g Protein, 5 g Carb, 167 mg Sodium

Green Olive Tapenade

Those who love olives will adore this spread, perfect for an hors d'oeuvre, served with fresh, raw vegetables. This is a quick and easy make-ahead dish.

1 cup pitted brine-cured green olives, such as Picholine

2 medium cloves garlic, roughly chopped

5 tablespoons extra-virgin olive oil

2 tablespoons chopped raw, unsalted almonds

1 tablespoon drained capers

1½ teaspoons fresh lemon juice

⅛ teaspoon kosher salt

⅛ teaspoon freshly ground black pepper

Small pinch of ground red pepper

Phase I: Detox
Gluten Free
Dairy Free
Quick
Vegetarian
Egg Free

Serves 6
Serving size: 2 tablespoons
Yield: ¾ cup
Prep time: 10 minutes
Cook time: none

Combine all ingredients in the bowl of a food processor fitted with a metal blade and process until smooth.

Nutritional Analysis

Per 2-tablespoon serving: 147 Calories, 15 g Fat, 2.0 g Sat, 0 mg Chol,

0 g Fiber, 1 g Protein, 2 g Carb, 237 mg Sodium

Creamy Chickpea Soup

Phase I: Detox
Gluten Free
Dairy Free
Vegetarian
(with vegetable broth)
Egg Free

Serves 4
Serving size: 1⅛ cups
Yield: 4½ cups
Prep time: 15 minutes
Cook time: 20 minutes

This easy, quick, creamy soup contains no cream, just puréed chickpeas, which lend a smooth richness of their own. The soup thickens as it sets, so you may need to add a little water when reheating.

6 tablespoons extra-virgin olive oil

¼ cup minced shallots

¼ cup minced celery

2 teaspoons minced garlic (1 medium clove)

½ teaspoon minced rosemary

4 cups low-sodium organic vegetable or chicken broth

2 (15-ounce) low-sodium cans or 3 cups cooked chickpeas, drained and rinsed

1 tablespoon low-sodium tomato paste

½ teaspoon kosher salt

1 teaspoon freshly ground black pepper

2 tablespoons snipped chives

Heat the extra-virgin olive oil in a medium saucepan over medium-high heat. Add the shallots and celery and cook for about 3 minutes, until the vegetables begin to soften. Add the garlic and rosemary and cook 30 seconds. Add the broth, chickpeas, tomato paste, salt, and pepper. Bring the soup to a simmer. Cook, uncovered, over medium-low heat for 10 to 15 minutes, until the chickpeas are soft.

When the soup is finished cooking, remove it from the heat and let cool slightly. Purée the soup in batches in a blender, returning the batches to a large saucepan. If the soup is too thick, add a little water. Serve garnished with the snipped chives.

Nutritional Analysis

Per 1⅛-cup serving: 395 Calories, 24 g Fat, 3.0 g Sat, 0 mg Chol,

8 g Fiber, 10 g Protein, 37 g Carb, 506 mg Sodium

Escarole and Rice Soup

This soup is real comfort food, thick and hearty. At the same time, the taste is delicate.

1 head of escarole (about 1 pound)

3 tablespoons extra-virgin olive oil

3 tablespoons minced shallots

3 tablespoons minced celery

½ teaspoon kosher salt

¾ cup brown rice

4 cups organic low-sodium chicken or vegetable broth

¼ teaspoon freshly ground black pepper

Phase I: Detox
Gluten Free
Dairy Free
Vegetarian (with vegetable broth)
Egg Free

Serves 6
Serving size: 1 cup
Yield: 6 cups
Prep time: 15 minutes
Cook time: 40 minutes

Remove any discolored or damaged outer leaves from the escarole. Wash the escarole thoroughly and cut crosswise into ribbons about ¾ inch thick.

Heat the extra-virgin olive oil in a large pan over medium-high heat. Add the shallots and celery and cook for 2 to 3 minutes, until the shallots are translucent. Add the salt. Add the rice and stir to coat it in the oil. Add the escarole and cook for about 5 minutes, stirring, until it wilts. Add the broth, bring to a simmer, and cook covered for about 35 minutes, or until the rice is tender. Stir in the black pepper.

Nutritional Analysis

Per 1-cup serving, 196 Calories, 9 g Fat, 2.1 g Sat, 6 mg Chol, 3 g Fiber, 7 g Protein, 21 g Carb, 333 mg Sodium

Gazpacho with Shrimp

Phase I: Detox
Gluten Free
Dairy Free
Egg Free

Serves 8
Serving size: 1 cup
Yield: 8 cups
Prep time: 45 minutes
Cook time: 10 minutes

The quintessential summer soup—gazpacho is best made when local tomatoes and vegetables are in season. If you make it in the wintertime, use ripe grape tomatoes. This gazpacho is easily made and can be refrigerated for up to a day in advance of serving.

4 cups diced tomatoes (about 4 large tomatoes)

1 cup diced red bell pepper (about 1 large pepper)

½ cup diced green bell pepper (about 1 small pepper)

½ cup diced red onion

1 tablespoon minced jalapeño pepper

1 large cucumber, peeled, seeded, and diced

1 tablespoon minced garlic (about 3 medium cloves)

¾ cup finely chopped cilantro

¼ cup fresh lime juice

3 cups low-sodium tomato juice

1 teaspoon freshly ground black pepper

½ recipe Seared Butterflied Shrimp (page 101)

Extra-virgin olive oil, for drizzling

8 chives, cut in ½-inch pieces

In a blender or food processor, mix the tomatoes, red pepper, green pepper, onion, jalapeño pepper, cucumber, garlic, cilantro, lime juice, tomato juice, and pepper until they are a souplike consistency. Refrigerate for at least 30 minutes before serving.

For each serving, slice 1 pan-seared shrimp into long strips and place the pieces overlapping on top of the gazpacho. Drizzle extra-virgin olive oil over the shrimp just before putting on the table. Garnish with the chive pieces.

Nutritional Analysis

Per 1-cup serving: 101 Calories, 3 g Fat, 0.5 g Sat, 42 mg Chol,

2.6 g Fiber, 7 g Protein, 13 g Carb, 355 mg Sodium

Ginger Carrot Soup

A dairy-free soup, this is made creamy with the addition of coconut milk. Fresh cilantro and sliced scallions enhance the visual appeal when used as a finishing touch just before serving.

2 tablespoons light sesame oil

1 large onion, peeled and diced (about 1 cup)

2 tablespoons minced ginger

1 medium clove garlic, minced (about 1 teaspoon)

2 pounds carrots, peeled and diced

4 cups organic low-sodium chicken or vegetable broth

¾ cup canned unsweetened lite coconut milk

½ teaspoon kosher salt

1 teaspoon fresh lime juice

¼ teaspoon Thai Kitchen Red Chili Paste

2 scallions, thinly sliced on the diagonal

¼ cup minced cilantro

Phase I: Detox
Gluten Free
Dairy Free
Vegetarian (with vegetable broth)
Egg Free

Serves 6
Serving size: 1 cup
Yield: 6 cups
Prep time: 40 minutes
Cook time: 30 minutes

Heat the sesame oil in a large pan over medium heat. Add the diced onion and ginger and cook for about 3 minutes, until the onion is translucent. Add the garlic and cook for 1 minute. Add the carrots and cook for 2 minutes. Add the broth, coconut milk, and salt. Cook for about 20 to 25 minutes, until the carrots are tender enough to pierce with a fork.

When the soup is finished cooking, remove it from the heat and cool slightly. Purée the soup in a blender, in batches, returning the puréed soup to a large saucepan. Add the lime juice and red chili paste. Taste and adjust seasonings if necessary. Just before serving, garnish the soup with the sliced scallion and cilantro.

Nutritional Analysis

Per 1-cup serving: 152 Calories, 7.5 g Fat, 6.4 g Sat, 17 mg Chol,

5 g Fiber, 6 g Protein, 17 g Carb, 435 mg Sodium

Lentil Soup

Phase I: Detox
Gluten Free
Dairy Free
Vegetarian (with vegetable stock)
Egg Free

Serves 6
Serving size: 1 cup
Yield: 6 cups
Prep time: 25 minutes
Cook time: 1 hour (25 minutes)

Earthy, satisfying, and hearty enough for a main course, thick, rich lentil soup is perfect for a cold winter day. If the soup becomes too thick, thin with a little water, chicken or vegetable stock, or broth.

3 tablespoons extra-virgin olive oil

½ cup diced leek (1½ ounces)

¼ cup minced shallots (about 1 ounce)

½ teaspoon minced garlic

1 cup diced carrots (about 1 large carrot)

½ cup diced celery

½ cup celery leaves

1 (15-ounce) can chopped tomatoes (about 1½ cups)

½ pound (2 cups) French green lentils, rinsed and picked over

5 cups organic low-sodium chicken or vegetable stock

1 multibranch sprig of thyme

¾ teaspoon kosher salt

½ teaspoon freshly ground black pepper

Heat the extra-virgin olive oil in a large saucepan over medium-high heat. Add the leek, shallots, and garlic. Cook, stirring, for about 3 minutes, until the shallots are translucent. Add the carrot, celery, and celery leaves. Cook for about 3 minutes, until the celery is softened.

Add the tomatoes, lentils, stock or broth, thyme, salt, and pepper. Bring to a simmer and cook, uncovered, until the lentils are soft, about 1 hour and 15 minutes. The cooking time of the lentils may vary. Remove the thyme sprig before serving.

Nutritional Analysis

Per 1-cup serving: 332 Calories, 10 g Fat, 2.0 g Sat, 7 mg Chol,

11 g Fiber, 19 g Protein, 43 g Carb, 593 mg Sodium

Three Mushroom Soup

Creamy in texture, this soup uses three varieties of mushrooms, which add an earthy depth of flavor.

2 tablespoons extra-virgin olive oil

1 medium leek, white and light green parts only, thoroughly washed and chopped (about 1 cup)

½ cup thinly sliced shallots

½ cup sliced celery

1 pound white button mushrooms, stems removed, cleaned and sliced

½ pound shiitake mushrooms, stems removed, cleaned and sliced

½ pound cremini mushroom, stems removed, cleaned and sliced

1 teaspoon chopped thyme

¾ teaspoon kosher salt

½ teaspoon freshly ground black pepper

5 cups organic low-sodium chicken or vegetable broth

3 tablespoons minced parsley

2 tablespoons snipped chives

Phase I: Detox
Gluten Free
Dairy Free
Vegetarian (with vegetable broth)
Egg Free

Serves 8
Serving size: 1 cup
Yield: 8 cups
Prep time: 30 minutes
Cook time: 45 minutes

Heat the extra-virgin olive oil in a large pan over medium heat. Add the leek, shallots, and celery and cook, stirring occasionally, for about 10 minutes, until softened. Add the mushrooms, thyme, salt, and pepper. Cook for about 10 minutes, until the mushrooms soften. Add the broth, cover the pan, and simmer for 20 minutes.

When the soup is finished cooking, remove it from the heat and cool slightly. Purée the soup in batches in a blender, returning the batches to a large saucepan. Stir in the parsley and gently heat the soup through. Serve garnished with the chives.

Nutritional Analysis

Per 1-cup serving: 93 Calories, 4 g Fat, 0.8 g Sat, 16 mg Chol, 1 g Fiber, 6 g Protein, 8 g Carb, 278 mg Sodium

Roasted Tomato Soup

Phase I: Detox
Gluten Free
Dairy Free
Vegetarion (with vegetable broth)
Egg Free

Serves 4
Serving size: 1 cup
Yield: 4 cups
Prep time: 20 minutes
Cook time: 50 minutes

This stunning, bright red-orange soup is thick and rich, with a slight smokiness from the roasted tomatoes and the paprika. If canned fire-roasted tomatoes are not available, substitute traditional canned whole tomatoes. The soup will be just as tasty, but not as smoky in flavor. Double-concentrated tomato paste is sold in a tube; if not available, substitute double the quantity of regular tomato paste.

2 tablespoons extra-virgin olive oil

½ cup chopped shallots

1 medium clove garlic, chopped

1 (28-ounce) can fire-roasted whole tomatoes, chopped

2 cups low-sodium organic chicken or vegetable broth

1 tablespoon double-concentrated tomato paste or 2 tablespoons regular tomato paste

½ teaspoon freshly ground black pepper

Pinch of ground red pepper

¼–½ teaspoon smoked Spanish paprika

1 small sprig of thyme

½ cup packed fresh basil leaves plus additional leaves for garnish

Heat the extra-virgin olive oil in a soup pot over medium heat. Add the shallots and cook for 3 to 5 minutes, until translucent. Add the garlic and cook until softened and fragrant, about 1 minute.

Stir in the tomatoes, broth, tomato paste, black pepper, red pepper, paprika, and thyme. Bring to a boil, reduce to a simmer, and cook for 35 minutes. Stir in the fresh basil leaves and simmer for 10 minutes. Remove from the heat and let cool slightly.

Purée the soup in a blender, in batches, returning the puréed soup to a large saucepan. Gently warm the soup if necessary before serving, garnished with the additional basil leaves.

Nutritional Analysis

Per 1-cup serving: 170 Calories, 7 g Fat, 1.2 g Sat, 3 mg Chol, 2 g Fiber, 6 g Protein, 21 g Carb, 518 mg Sodium

Split Green Pea Soup

Thick and hearty, this filling soup makes a nice main course for lunch or supper.

2 tablespoons extra-virgin olive oil

½ cup chopped onion

1 pound (2 cups) green split peas

1½ cups chopped carrot

1 cup chopped russet potato (about 1 medium potato)

½ cup chopped celery

1 medium clove garlic, chopped

8 cups vegetable broth

¼ cup chopped parsley

½ teaspoon minced thyme

½ teaspoon minced oregano

1 bay leaf

½ teaspoon kosher salt

¾ teaspoon freshly ground black pepper

2 tablespoons low-sodium tomato paste

1 teaspoon fresh lemon juice

Phase I: Detox
Gluten Free
Dairy Free
Vegetarian
Egg Free

Serves 8
Serving size: 1 cup
Yield: 8 cups
Prep time: 15 minutes,
plus 15 minutes to purée
and finish
Cook time: 65 minutes

Heat the extra-virgin olive oil in a large saucepan over medium heat. Add the onion and cook, stirring, for about 3 minutes, until translucent. Add the peas, carrot, potato, celery, and garlic; stir to coat in the oil. Add the broth, parsley, thyme, oregano, bay leaf, salt, and pepper. Bring to a boil, reduce to a simmer, and cook, uncovered, for 50 to 60 minutes, or until all the vegetables are soft. Periodically skim off the foam that rises to the top of the soup during cooking.

When the soup is finished cooking, allow to cool slightly. Remove and discard the bay leaf. Pass the soup through a food mill and return to a pan. Add the tomato paste and lemon juice and heat through over low heat. For smoother soup, purée in batches in a blender. If the soup becomes too thick, stir in a little water and reheat.

Nutritional Analysis

Per 1-cup serving: 300 Calories, 6 g Fat, 1.1 g Sat, 25 mg Chol, 16 g Fiber, 20 g Protein, 44 g Carb, 316 mg Sodium

Black Bean Soup

Phase I: Detox
Gluten Free
Dairy Free
Vegetarian
(with vegetable broth)
Egg Free

Serves 4
Serving size: 1¼ cups
Yield: 5 cups
Prep time: 20 minutes
Cook time: 35 minutes

This quick, easy soup is accented by the colors of the red pepper and cilantro. It is thick and lends itself to many garnishes, such as diced avocado or red onion. If desired, increase the jalapeño pepper for more heat.

2 tablespoons extra-virgin olive oil

½ cup chopped onion

2 teaspoons minced garlic

4 cups cooked or low-sodium canned black beans, rinsed and drained

2½ cups organic low-sodium vegetable or chicken broth

1 cup chopped fresh tomatoes

½ cup diced red bell pepper

2 teaspoons minced jalapeño pepper

2 tablespoons molasses

2 teaspoons minced oregano

1½ teaspoons ground cumin

½ teaspoon ground coriander

½ teaspoon kosher salt

½ teaspoon freshly ground black pepper

2 tablespoons minced cilantro

2 teaspoons fresh lime juice

Heat the extra-virgin olive oil in a large Dutch oven or soup pot over medium-high heat. Add the onion and garlic and cook for 3 minutes, until softened. Stir in the beans, broth, tomatoes, red pepper, jalapeño pepper, molasses, oregano, cumin, coriander, salt, and black pepper. Bring to a boil, reduce the heat to medium-low, and simmer for 30 minutes, until the vegetables are soft. Stir in the cilantro and lime juice.

Nutritional Analysis

Per 1¼-cup serving: 340 Calories, 8 g Fat, 1.3 g Sat, 3 mg Chol,

14 g Fiber, 18 g Protein, 51 g Carb, 568 mg Sodium

Creamy Cauliflower Soup

The fresh herbs add a nice flavor and color to this smooth and creamy soup.

2 tablespoons extra-virgin olive oil

2 small leeks, white and pale green parts only, thoroughly washed and chopped (about 1¼ cups)

1 medium head cauliflower, broken into florets and thinly sliced

5 cups organic low-sodium vegetable or chicken broth or stock

1¼ teaspoons kosher salt

½ teaspoon freshly ground black pepper

1 tablespoon minced parsley

Pinch of ground red pepper

1 tablespoon snipped chives

Phase I: Detox
Gluten Free
Dairy Free
Vegetarian (with vegetable broth or stock)
Egg Free

Serves 6
Serving size: 1 cup
Yield: 6 cups
Prep time: 30 minutes
Cook time: 30 minutes

Heat the extra-virgin olive oil in a large saucepan over medium heat. Add the leeks and cook, stirring, for about 5 minutes, until soft. Add the cauliflower, broth, salt, and black pepper and bring to a boil. Reduce the heat, then cover and simmer for 20 to 25 minutes, until the vegetables are soft.

Let the soup cool slightly. Purée the soup, in batches, in a blender until smooth. Return the soup to the pan and add the parsley and ground red pepper. Heat the soup through and garnish with chives before serving.

Nutritional Analysis

Per 1-cup serving: 106 Calories, 6 g Fat, 1.2 g Sat, 5 mg Chol, 3 g Fiber, 7 g Protein, 9 g Carb, 285 mg Sodium

Asian Vegetable Salad

Phase I: Detox
Gluten Free
Dairy Free
Quick
Vegetarian
Egg Free

Serves 4
Serving size: 1 cup
Yield: 4 cups
Prep time: 30 minutes
Cook time: minimal

The dressing is well balanced with salty, sweet, and sour tastes. This salad is a perfect accompaniment for Soy-Marinated Tofu (page 118), or any grilled or roasted meat.

¼ pound snow peas (generous 1 cup), stem ends trimmed and strings removed

2 cups shredded Napa or Savoy cabbage

⅓ cup julienne carrot

⅓ cup julienne red bell pepper

⅓ cup julienne cucumber

3 tablespoons minced scallion (about 1 medium scallion)

2 tablespoons minced cilantro

1 tablespoon minced mint

3 tablespoons light sesame oil

1 tablespoon low-sodium wheat-free tamari

1 tablespoon rice wine vinegar

1 tablespoon fresh lime juice

¼ teaspoon freshly ground black pepper

Bring a large pot of salted water to a boil. Add the snow peas and cook for 30 seconds. Drain and immediately place in a bowl of ice water. Remove the snow peas from the ice water and pat dry.

Mix together the snow peas, cabbage, carrot, red pepper, cucumber, scallion, cilantro, and mint.

Whisk together the sesame oil, tamari, rice wine vinegar, lime juice, and pepper in a small bowl. Pour the dressing over the vegetables and mix thoroughly.

Nutritional Analysis

Per 1-cup serving: 125 Calories, 11 g Fat, 1.5 g Sat, 0 mg Chol,

2 g Fiber, 1.9 g Protein, 6.4 g Carb, 164 mg Sodium

Asian Bean Salad with Tahini Dressing

Tahini is a Middle Eastern sauce that has a delicious tang. Added to a salad like this it makes a light, refreshing dish full of flavor.

Phase I: Detox
Gluten Free
Dairy Free
Quick
Vegetarian
Egg Free

Serves 2
Serving size: 3½ cups
Yield: 7 cups
Prep time: 15 minutes
Cook time: none

Tahini Dressing

¼ cup tahini

2 tablespoons extra-virgin olive oil

1 tablespoon minced garlic

2 tablespoons freshly squeezed lemon juice

Pinch kosher salt

Dash freshly cracked black pepper

Asian Bean Salad

4 cups fresh baby spinach

¼ cup chopped scallions

½ cup snow peas, strings removed

1 cup bean sprouts, rinsed and drained

1 cup drained canned adzuki beans

In a small bowl, whisk together the tahini, olive oil, garlic, lemon juice, salt, and pepper. Place the spinach, scallions, snow peas, bean sprouts, and beans in a large salad bowl. Pour the tahini dressing over the vegetable mixture and toss together to coat. Serve.

Nutritional Analysis

Per 3½-cup serving: 426 Calories, 28 g Fat, 4.2 g Sat, 0 mg Chol,

12 g Fiber, 13 g Protein, 35 g Carb, 160 mg Sodium

Green Bean and Tomato Salad with Toasted Pumpkin Seeds

Phase I: Detox
Gluten Free
Dairy Free
Vegetarian
Egg Free

Serves 6
Serving size: ½ cup
Yield: 3 cups
Prep time: 30 minutes
Cook time: 10 minutes

The lime in the dressing is pronounced and is complemented by the creaminess of the avocado.

¼ cup hulled raw, unsalted pumpkin seeds

1 pound green beans, stem ends trimmed, cut in half diagonally

1 cup diced tomato

¼ cup thinly sliced small red onion

2 teaspoons minced oregano

3 tablespoons minced cilantro

1 teaspoon minced garlic

½ teaspoon ground cumin

½ teaspoon kosher salt

½ teaspoon freshly ground black pepper

½ teaspoon lime zest

2½ tablespoons fresh lime juice

6 tablespoons extra-virgin olive oil

½ small avocado, peeled, pitted, and diced (about ¼ cup)

Toast the pumpkin seeds in a small skillet over medium heat for 3 to 5 minutes, until they are puffed up. Stir frequently and watch closely to prevent burning. When toasted, remove the seeds to a plate.

Bring 6 cups of water to boil in a medium pan. Add the beans. Cook for about 3 minutes, until the beans are crisp-tender. Drain, and immediately transfer the beans to a bowl of ice water to stop the cooking. Drain and shake dry. Place the beans in a large bowl with the tomato, onion, oregano, and cilantro.

In a small bowl, combine the garlic, cumin, salt, pepper, lime zest, and lime juice. Slowly whisk in the extra-virgin olive oil until slightly thickened. Pour the dressing over the beans. Stir in the avocado. Add the pumpkin seeds and combine. Adjust the seasoning and serve.

Nutritional Analysis

Per ½-cup serving: 221 Calories, 20 g Fat, 2.9 g Sat, 0 mg Chol,

4 g Fiber, 4 g Protein, 10 g Carb, 169 mg Sodium

Black Bean Confetti Salad

A colorful, naturally sweet, antioxidant rich salad.

One 15-ounce can black beans, rinsed and drained

1 cup frozen organic corn, thawed and drained

12 cherry or grape tomatoes, halved

½ cup chopped scallions

2 cloves garlic, pressed

½ cup diced red bell pepper

¼ cup chopped cilantro

2 tablespoons extra-virgin olive oil

3 tablespoons freshly squeezed lime juice

¼ teaspoon ground cumin

Phase I: Detox
Gluten Free
Dairy Free
Quick
Vegetarian
Egg Free

Serves 2
Serving size: 1½ cups
Yield: 3 cups
Prep time: 15 minutes
(plus marinating time)
Cook time: none

Mix all the ingredients in a large bowl, cover, and let marinate in the refrigerator for a few hours before serving.

Nutritional Analysis

Per 1½-cup serving: 412 Calories, 15 g Fat, 2.2 g Sat, 0 mg Chol,

18 g Fiber, 18 g Protein, 57 g Carb, 110 mg Sodium

Mint-Scented Salad with Lime-Rice Wine Vinaigrette

Phase I: Detox
Gluten Free
Dairy Free
Quick
Vegetarian
Egg Free

Serves 4
Serving size: 2 cups
Yield: 8 cups
Prep time: 10 minutes
Cook time: none

Easy to prepare, this refreshing salad is especially good with Scallops poached in Thai Coconut Curry Broth (page 106).

8 cups Boston lettuce, washed and cut into bite-size pieces
4 scallions, thinly sliced on the diagonal
½ hothouse cucumber, unpeeled and thinly sliced
1 teaspoon chopped mint
1 recipe Lime–Rice Wine Vinaigrette (page 175)

Mix the lettuce, scallions, cucumber, and mint. Toss with the Lime–Rice Wine Vinaigrette.

Nutritional Analysis

Per 2-cup serving: 159 Calories, 14 g Fat, 2.0 g Sat, 0 mg Chol, 2 g Fiber, 2 g Protein, 7 g Carb, 511 mg Sodium

Romaine and Avocado Salad with Toasted Pumpkin Seeds

This filling salad is crunchy with pumpkin seeds and creamy with avocado, with a Southwestern twist from the Spicy Cilantro-Lime Vinaigrette (page 178).

½ cup hulled raw, unsalted pumpkin seeds

1 medium head Romaine lettuce, cut into bite-size pieces (about 8 cups)

1 cup chopped tomato

2 large scallions, thinly sliced on the diagonal (about ½ cup)

½ medium red or yellow bell pepper, cored, seeded, and cut in thin strips (about ½ cup)

1 recipe Spicy Cilantro-Lime Vinaigrette (page 178)

1 large avocado, peeled, pitted, and diced

Phase I: Detox
Gluten Free
Dairy Free
Quick
Vegetarian
Egg Free

Serves 6
Serving size: 1½ cups
Yield: 9 cups
Prep time: 20 minutes
Cook time: none

Toast the pumpkin seeds in a small skillet over medium-low heat for about 3 to 4 minutes, until puffed and lightly browned. Stir frequently and watch closely to prevent burning. When toasted, remove the seeds to a plate to cool.

In a large bowl, combine the lettuce, tomato, scallions, peppers, and toasted pumpkin seeds. Add the dressing and toss to combine. Add the avocado and toss again.

Nutritional Analysis

Per 1½-cup serving: 331 Calories, 31 g Fat, 4.5 g Sat, 0 mg Chol, 5 g Fiber, 6 g Protein, 11 g Carb, 255 mg Sodium

Curried Waldorf Salad

Phase I: Detox
Gluten Free
Dairy Free
Quick
Vegetarian
Egg Free

Serves 2
Prep time: 15 minutes
Cook time: none

A nutty, dairy-free version of a traditional favorite.

¼ cup chopped walnuts

1 large Red Delicious or Gala apple, skin on, cored and diced

1 cup extra-firm tofu, drained well and cut into 1-inch cubes

½ cup chopped celery

½ tablespoon flaxseed, ground

½ teaspoon grated fresh ginger

½ teaspoon curry powder

1 tablespoon walnut oil

1 head endive, separated and washed

Sprinkle nuts in a single layer on a cookie sheet and toast at 350 degrees F. for 10 to 15 minutes, stirring occasionally.

In a large bowl, combine the apple, tofu, celery, walnuts, flaxseed, ginger, curry powder, and oil. Arrange endive in layers on salad plates. Spoon the apple-tofu mixture on the endive and serve.

Nutritional Analysis

Per serving: 286 Calories, 16 g Fat, 2.5 g Sat, 0 mg Chol, 12 g Fiber, 16 g Protein, 28 g Carb, 88 mg Sodium

Endive and Walnut Salad

This classic French salad contrasts flavors and textures beautifully.

1¾ pounds Belgian endive (about 6 medium to large heads)

¾ cup chopped raw, unsalted walnuts (about 3 ounces)

½ cup extra-virgin olive oil

3 tablespoons fresh lemon juice

½ teaspoon kosher salt

½ teaspoon freshly ground pepper

Phase I: Detox
Gluten Free
Dairy Free
Quick
Vegetarian
Egg Free

Serves 6
Serving size: 1 cup
Yield: 6 cups
Prep time: 20 minutes
Cook time: 10 minutes

Slice the endive vertically into strips about ½ inch wide.

Toast the walnuts in a small skillet over medium heat. Stir the nuts for about 10 minutes, until lightly toasted. Watch carefully, as nuts can burn easily. Remove to a plate to cool.

In a large bowl, combine the extra-virgin olive oil, lemon juice, salt, and pepper.

Toss the endive strips with the dressing. Divide the endive onto 6 plates. Top with the toasted walnuts.

Nutritional Analysis

Per 1-cup serving: 285 Calories, 28 g Fat, 3.5 g Sat, 0 mg Chol, 5 g Fiber, 3 g Protein, 8 g Carb, 163 mg Sodium

Mediterranean Chopped Salad

Phase I: Detox
Gluten Free
Dairy Free
Quick
Vegetarian
Egg Free

Serves 4
Serving size: 1¾ cups
Yield: 7 cups
Prep time: 30 minutes
Cook time: none

Simple and refreshing, this is a wonderful accompaniment to dishes like Middle Eastern Lamb Patties (page 110).

½ cup thinly sliced red onion

1 large romaine lettuce heart, chopped (about 4 cups)

1 cup grape tomatoes, cut in half (about 6 ounces)

1 medium green pepper, cored, seeded, and cut into ¾-inch pieces

½ hothouse cucumber, cut in half lengthwise and sliced

½ cup pitted Kalamata olives, halved

1 teaspoon minced oregano

1 recipe of Basic Vinaigrette (page 174)

Soak the red onion in a small bowl of ice water for about 10 minutes. Drain and pat dry.

Place the onion in a large salad bowl and combine with the chopped lettuce, tomatoes, green pepper, cucumber, olives, and oregano. Toss with the vinaigrette.

Nutritional Analysis

Per 1¾-cup serving: 244 Calories, 23 fg Fat, 3.2 g Sat, 0 mg Chol,

3 g Fiber, 2 g Protein, 9 g Carb, 395 mg Sodium

Orange and Red Onion Salad with Fennel

A lovely salad to make in midwinter, when citrus fruit is at its peak.

Phase I: Detox
Gluten Free
Dairy Free
Quick
Vegetarian
Egg Free

Serves 4
Prep time: 15 minutes
Cook time: none

3 tablespoons extra-virgin olive oil

1½ tablespoons fresh lemon juice

¼ teaspoon kosher salt

½ teaspoon coarsely ground black pepper

2 large navel oranges

½ cup very thinly sliced fennel

¼ cup very thinly sliced red onion

3 tablespoons chopped mint

8 brine-cured black olives, such as Kalamata, pitted and quartered

Whisk together the extra–virgin olive oil, lemon juice, salt, and pepper.

Peel the oranges, removing all the white pith, and cut them horizontally into ¼-inch-thick slices. Arrange the oranges on a platter or in a shallow dish and pour 3 tablespoons of the dressing over them.

Toss the fennel, red onion, and mint with the remainder of the dressing. Arrange the fennel mixture on top of the orange slices. Garnish with the olives.

Nutritional Analysis

Per serving: 168 Calories, 13 g Fat, 1.7 g Sat, 0 mg Chol, 3 g Fiber, 1 g Protein, 14 g Carb, 249 mg Sodium

Tricolor Salad

Phase I: Detox
Gluten Free
Dairy Free
Quick
Vegetarian
Egg Free

Serves 6
Serving size: 1⅔ cups
Yield: 10 cups
Prep time: 10 minutes
Cook time: none

A nice twist on a traditional salad, this mix has a pleasing texture and crunch, especially from the walnuts. The pomegranate vinaigrette is sweeter than traditional red wine vinaigrette, and provides a pleasing balance for the bitter greens.

½ cup chopped raw, unsalted walnuts

4 cups baby arugula (about 4 ounces)

2 small Belgian endive, cut lengthwise into ½-inch strips (about 3 cups)

½ small head radicchio, sliced (about 3 cups)

1 recipe Pomegranate Vinaigrette (page 174)

Toast the walnuts in a small skillet over medium heat for about 5 minutes, until slightly darker in color. Stir frequently and watch closely to prevent burning. When toasted, remove the walnuts to a plate to cool.

Place the toasted walnuts, arugula, endive, and radicchio in a large bowl and toss with the pomegranate vinaigrette.

Nutritional Analysis

Per 1⅔-cup serving: 223 Calories, 21 g Fat, 2.6 g Sat, 0 mg Chol,

3 g Fiber, 3 g Protein, 8 g Carb, 182 mg Sodium

Cashew Chicken Salad

The combination of cashews with citrus fruit gives this dish nutty and naturally sweet flavor that is nicely complimented by the slightly spicy tang of ginger: a classically Asian combination of flavors.

4 ounces dry rice noodles (or 2 cups cooked)

Dressing

1 tablespoon cashew butter

1 tablespoon plain unseasoned rice vinegar

2 tablespoons freshly squeezed lime juice

1 teaspoon minced fresh ginger

1 tablespoon minced garlic

1 teaspoon lime zest

Salad

1 cup cooked diced chicken

2 cups shredded Napa Cabbage

2 sliced scallions

1 cup sliced carrots

½ cup sliced red bell pepper

1 fresh orange, cut into chunks

Garnish

1 tablespoon chopped fresh cilantro

3 tablespoons chopped cashews

Phase I: Detox
Gluten Free
Dairy Free
Quick
Vegetarian
Egg Free

Serves: 2
Serving Size: 2 cups
Yield: 4 cups
Prep Time: 20 minutes
Cook Time: 10 minutes

Prepare the rice noodles according to package directions.

Combine cashew butter, rice vinegar, lime juice, ginger, garlic, and lime zest in a small bowl and stir vigorously until smooth.

Place salad ingredients in a medium salad bowl along with the rice noodles and mix well. Pour dressing over the vegetables and noodles. Garnish with fresh chopped cilantro and cashews.

Nutritional Analysis

Per 2-cup serving: 441 Calories, 11 g Fat, 2 g Sat, 68 mg Chol, 9 g Fiber, 35 g Protein, 53 g Carb, 191 mg Sodium

Sunflower Tofu Spinach Salad with Pomegranate Dressing

Phase I: Detox
Serves: 2
Prep time: 10 minutes
Cook Time: None

Baby spinach with a slightly sweet dressing is a classic combination. This variant uses pomegranate and adds crunch (as well as protein) through the use of sunflowers.

6 cups fresh baby spinach

3 thinly sliced radishes

½ thinly sliced small red onion

¼ cup grated carrots

¼ cup raw sunflower seeds, shelled

8 ounces baked and seasoned tofu, cut into 1" cubes

1 medium pear, sliced

½ cup Pomegranate Dressing I (recipe follows)

Combine all salad ingredients in a large mixing bowl. Pour dressing over top. Toss together and mix well. Serve.

Nutritional Analysis

Per serving: 258 Calories, 14.2 g Fat, 2.1 g Sat, 0 mg Chol, 8 g Fiber, 12 g Protein, 25 g Carb, 78 mg Sodium

Pomegranate Dressing (I)

⅓ cup extra-virgin olive oil

⅓ cup freshly squeezed lemon juice

4 tablespoons pure pomegranate juice

1 tablespoon Dijon mustard

1 tablespoon pomegranate molasses

pinch Kosher salt

dash freshly ground black pepper

Phase I: Detox
Serves 8
Serving size: 2 tablespoons
Yield: 1 cup
Prep time: 5 minutes

Combine all ingredients in a small bowl and mix until thoroughly blended.

Nutritional Analysis

Per 2-tablespoon serving: 90 Calories, 8 g Fat, 0 mg Chol, 0 g Fiber, 0 g Protein, 5 g Carb, 35 mg Sodium

Totals: 348 Calories, 22 g Fat, 0 mg Chol, 8 g Fiber, 12 g Protein, 30 g Carb, 113 mg Sodium

Asian Chicken Salad

Phase I: Detox
Gluten Free
Dairy Free
Egg Free

Serves 4
Serving size: 1 cup salad
plus ¼ cup dressing
Yield: 4 cups salad plus
1 cup dressing
Prep time: 40 minutes
Cook time: minimal

With a rich dressing made from tahini (sesame seed paste), this colorful, filling salad is perfect for lunch, picnics, or as part of a dinner party buffet.

2 ounces snow peas, strings removed (generous ½ cup)

3 cups cooked chicken breast, shredded

½ cup thinly sliced red bell pepper

½ cup julienne carrots

¼ cup thinly sliced scallions (about 2 scallions, sliced on the diagonal)

1 cup Tahini Dressing (page 173)

2 tablespoons black sesame seeds

Bring a large pan of salted water to a boil. Drop in the snow peas and cook for 30 seconds. Drain, and immediately place in a bowl of ice water to stop the cooking. Drain again, and cut the snow peas on the diagonal into thin slices.

Place the snow peas in a large bowl. Add the chicken, red pepper, carrot, and scallion, and stir to combine.

Stir 1 cup of the dressing into the chicken mixture. Add more dressing if desired. Garnish the chicken salad with the sesame seeds before serving.

Nutritional Analysis

Per 1 cup salad and ¼ cup dressing: 533 Calories, 39 g Fat, 5.8 g Sat, 90 mg Chol,

3 g Fiber, 40 g Protein, 8.5 g Carb, 660 mg Sodium

Grilled Shrimp Brochettes

In this easy and delicious dish, the herb and lemon flavors pair well with the fresh shrimp and the red pepper flakes add a slight kick of heat. Made on small skewers, these make tasty hors d'oeuvres. If using bamboo skewers, soak the skewers in a shallow dish of water for one hour before threading with the shrimp.

Phase I: Detox
Gluten Free
Dairy Free
Quick
Egg Free

Serves 4
Serving size: 5 to 6 shrimp
Prep time: 10 minutes
Cook time: 4 minutes

¼ cup extra-virgin olive oil

2 teaspoons minced oregano

2 teaspoons minced parsley

1 teaspoon minced garlic

1 teaspoon lemon zest

½ teaspoon crushed red pepper flakes

½ teaspoon kosher salt

½ teaspoon freshly ground black pepper

1 pound large (21 to 25 count) shrimp, peeled and deveined

Lemon wedges for garnish

Mix together the extra-virgin olive oil, oregano, parsley, garlic, lemon zest, crushed red pepper flakes, salt, and pepper. Toss the shrimp in the olive oil and herbs. Cover and refrigerate for 1 hour.

Thread the shrimp on 4 skewers, placing 5 to 6 shrimp on each skewer.

Preheat an outdoor grill or an indoor grill pan over medium–high heat. If using a grill pan, brush with 1 teaspoon of extra-virgin olive oil before heating. Grill the shrimp for 2 minutes on each side.

Serve with the lemon wedges.

Nutritional Analysis

Per brochette: 248 Calories, 16 g Fat, 2.3 g Sat, 172 mg Chol, 0 g Fiber, 23 g Pro, 1 g Carb, 409 mg Sodium

Pan-Browned Tilapia

Phase I: Detox
Gluten Free
Dairy Free
Quick
Egg Free

Serves 4
Serving size: 6 ounces
Yield: 4 (6-ounce) fillets
Prep time: 5 minutes
Cook time: 5 minutes

Crispy on the outside, flaky, white, and tender on the inside, this quick and easy fish has a lemony taste.

4 (6-ounce) tilapia fillets
½ teaspoon kosher salt
¼ teaspoon freshly ground black pepper
¼ cup chickpea or soy flour
5 tablespoons extra-virgin olive oil
¼ cup fresh lemon juice
3 tablespoons finely chopped parsley
Lemon wedges for garnish

Pat the fish dry with paper towels, and season both sides with the salt and pepper. Dredge the fish in the flour, shaking off any excess.

Heat 3 tablespoons of extra-virgin olive oil in a large skillet or sauté pan over medium-high heat. Add the fillets in a single layer and cook, in batches if necessary, for about 2 minutes on each side, until brown on the outside and flaky but moist on the inside. Transfer to a platter and keep warm.

Heat the remaining 2 tablespoons of extra-virgin olive oil in the pan over high heat. Add the lemon juice and parsley and cook for 30 seconds, scraping any browned bits off of the bottom of the pan. Pour the pan sauce over the fillets and serve. Garnish with lemon wedges.

Nutritional Analysis

Per 6-ounce fillet: 363 Calories, 21 g Fat, 3.5 g Sat, 85 mg Chol,

0.8 g Fiber, 35 g Protein, 10 g Carb, 330 mg Sodium

Pan-Seared Halibut

Searing the fish in a heavy skillet creates a beautiful brown, crunchy crust using simple ingredients—salt, pepper, and olive oil. The fillet is delicious on its own or served with a squeeze of fresh lemon.

4 (6-ounce) skinless halibut fillets

½ teaspoon kosher salt

½ teaspoon finely ground black pepper

2 tablespoons extra-virgin olive oil

Lemon wedges

Preheat the oven to 400 degrees F.

Season the fish on both sides with salt and pepper.

Heat the extra-virgin olive oil in an ovenproof skillet over high heat until smoking. Add the fillets and cook for 3 minutes on each side. Transfer the pan to the oven and continue cooking for 3 more minutes, or until cooked through.

Serve with the lemon wedges.

Phase I: Detox
Gluten Free
Dairy Free
Quick
Egg Free

Serves 4
Serving size: 6 ounces
Yield: 4 (6-ounce) fillets
Prep time: 5 minutes
Cook time: 10 minutes

Nutritional Analysis

Per 6-ounce fillet: 250 Calories, 11 g Fat, 1.5 g Sat, 54 mg Chol,

0 g Fiber, 36 g Protein, 0 g Carb, 394 mg Sodium

Roasted Shrimp

Phase I: Detox
Gluten Free
Dairy Free
Quick
Egg Free

Serves 4
Serving size: 5 to 6 shrimp
Yield: 1 pound large shrimp
Prep time: 5 minutes
Cook time: 25 minutes

A different way to prepare shrimp, roasting results in plump, tasty shrimp with no dryness. Very little olive oil is absorbed during roasting. Serve as a first course or as an hors d'oeuvre.

1 pound large (21 to 25 count) shrimp, peeled and deveined, tails left on if desired
¼ cup extra-virgin olive oil
¼ teaspoon kosher salt
Pinch of crushed red pepper flakes

Preheat the oven to 250 degrees F.

Place the shrimp in a baking dish just big enough to hold them in a single layer. Toss with the extra-virgin olive oil, salt, and crushed red pepper.

Roast the shrimp for about 25 minutes, until pink and firm to the touch, turning them twice during cooking.

Nutritional Analysis
Per 6-shrimp serving: 152 Calories, 5 g Fat, 0.9 g Sat, 172 mg Chol,
0 g Fiber, 23 g Protein, 1 g Carb, 288 mg Sodium

Seared Butterflied Shrimp

Simply delicious, quick and easy, this shrimp is great served alone with a squeeze of fresh lemon. Plan on three to four jumbo shrimp per person for a main course.

1 pound jumbo (16 to 20 count) shrimp, peeled and deveined

3 tablespoons extra-virgin olive oil

½ teaspoon kosher salt

¼ to ½ teaspoon crushed red pepper flakes

Fresh lemon wedges

Using a small paring knife, cut along the back of the shrimp, keeping the shrimp in one piece and not cutting all the way through to the other side. Open the shrimp and press flat. Toss with the extra-virgin olive oil, salt, and red pepper flakes.

Heat a large skillet over high heat, until very hot. Place the shrimp in the pan, in a single layer, and avoid crowding them. Cook for 2 minutes, then turn the shrimp, pressing them against the bottom of the pan to keep flat. Cook for 1 more minute.

Serve with lemon wedges.

Phase I: Detox
Gluten Free
Dairy Free
Quick
Egg Free

Serves 4
Serving size: 3 to 4 jumbo shrimp
Yield: 1 pound jumbo shrimp
Prep time: 10 minutes
Cook time: 2 to 3 minutes per batch

Nutritional Analysis

Per 4-ounce (3 to 4 shrimp) serving: 180 Calories, 11 g Fat, 1.7 g Sat, 168 mg Chol,

0 g Fiber, 18 g Protein, 0 g Carb, 433 mg Sodium

Spanish-Style Shrimp with Lemon and Garlic

Phase I: Detox
Gluten Free
Dairy Free
Quick
Egg Free

Serves 4 as an appetizer,
or 2 as a main course
Serving size: 7 to 8 shrimp
as appetizer, 14 to 15
shrimp as main course
Prep time: 15 minutes
Cook time: 10 minutes

This garlicky shrimp has an authentic taste found in traditional Spanish-style shrimp. Garlic is the predominant flavor, complemented by the Spanish paprika and red pepper flakes. Serve over steamed brown rice for a gluten-free meal.

4 tablespoons extra-virgin olive oil
6 medium cloves garlic, sliced
1 pound medium (31 to 35 per pound) shrimp, peeled and deveined
¼ teaspoon crushed red pepper flakes
¼ teaspoon Spanish paprika
1 small bay leaf
2 tablespoons fresh lemon juice
¼ cup minced parsley

Heat the extra-virgin olive oil in a medium skillet over medium heat. Add the garlic and cook until golden.

Add the shrimp, red pepper flakes, paprika, and bay leaf. Cook, stirring, for about 3 minutes, until the shrimp turns pink and is cooked throughout. Stir in the lemon juice.

Remove from the heat, add the minced parsley, and serve.

Nutritional Analysis

Per 4-ounce (7 to 8 shrimp) serving: 221 Calories, 15 g Fat, 2.2 g Sat, 168 mg Chol,

0 g Fiber, 18 g Protein, 2 g Carb, 196 mg Sodium

Steamed Mussels in Saffron Fennel Broth

Mussels steam beautifully in this golden broth, flavorful with saffron, carrots, and shallots. Serve this with a spoon, so that the broth can be eaten like soup.

2 pounds mussels, washed and beards removed

3 tablespoons extra-virgin olive oil

½ cup thinly sliced shallot

3 medium cloves garlic, thinly sliced

¼ small fennel bulb, cut in matchsticks (about ½ cup)

1 small carrot, cut in matchsticks (about ½ cup)

½ cup chopped fresh tomatoes

¼ teaspoon saffron threads, crumbled

1 sprig of thyme

½ teaspoon kosher salt

½ teaspoon freshly ground black pepper

1 cup water

¼ cup chopped parsley

Phase I: Detox
Gluten Free
Dairy Free
Egg Free

Serves 4
Serving size: ½ pound mussels
Yield: 2 pounds mussels
Prep time: 20 minutes
Cook time: 20 minutes

Discard any mussels that are open, have broken shells, or do not close when tapped with your finger.

Heat the extra-virgin olive oil in a large stockpot or Dutch oven over medium heat. Add the shallot and cook until soft and translucent, about 2 minutes. Add the garlic and cook for 1 minute more. Stir in the fennel, carrot, tomatoes, saffron, thyme, salt, and pepper. Cook, stirring, for 3 to 4 minutes, until the vegetables begin to soften. Add the water and bring to a boil. Reduce the heat and simmer the broth for 5 minutes.

Lay the mussels in the broth. Cover the pot and cook for about 4 minutes, or until the mussels open. Discard any mussels that do not open. Add the parsley and cook, stirring, for about 1 minute.

Serve the mussels in bowls with the broth and vegetables.

Nutritional Analysis

Per ½-pound serving: 240 Calories, 13 g Fat, 2.0 g Sat, 36 mg Chol, 1 g Fiber, 17 g Protein, 13 g Carb, 646 mg Sodium

Asian Spice-Rubbed Scallops with Sesame Dressing

Phase I: Detox
Gluten Free
Dairy Free
Quick
Egg Free

Serves 4
Serving size: 3 scallops
plus 2 tablespoons
dressing
Yield: 12 scallops plus
½ cup dressing
Prep time: 15 minutes
Cook time: 5 minutes

This dish is easy and fast, but also very elegant and delicious. The dressing is slightly sweet with a hint of soy and ginger, and it pairs beautifully with the spice rub. Serve with sautéed or stir-fried bok choy and steamed brown rice.

2 tablespoons rice wine vinegar

1 tablespoon fresh lime juice

2 teaspoons low-sodium wheat-free tamari

¾ teaspoon minced fresh ginger

3 tablespoons light sesame oil

1 tablespoon chopped cilantro

2 teaspoons ground cumin

2 teaspoons ground star anise

1 teaspoon ground coriander

½ teaspoon kosher salt

½ teaspoon ground ginger

½ teaspoon freshly ground Szechwan or black peppercorns

2 tablespoons extra-virgin olive oil

1 pound (about 12) large sea scallops

In a medium bowl, mix together the rice wine vinegar, lime juice, tamari, and fresh ginger. Slowly whisk in the sesame oil until well blended and slightly thickened. Stir in the cilantro.

For the spice rub, in a small bowl, mix together the cumin, star anise, coriander, salt, ginger, and pepper.

Heat the extra-virgin olive oil in a large skillet over medium–high heat. Coat the scallops on 1 side with the spice mixture. Place in the hot skillet, spice side down, and cook for 2 minutes. Gently turn the scallops with a spatula or tongs and cook on the other side for about 2 more minutes, until browned and just cooked through. Cooking time will vary with the size of the scallops.

To serve, divide the scallops into 4 portions and top each portion with 2 tablespoons of the dressing.

Nutritional Analysis

Per 3 scallops plus 2 tablespoons dressing serving: 285 Calories, 19 g Fat, 2.5 g Sat,

37 mg Chol, 0 g Fiber, 19 g Protein, 9.4 g Carb, 595 mg Sodium

Lobster Fra Diavalo

These succulent pieces of lobster in a somewhat spicy sauce are best served over a cooked whole grain such as brown rice.

3 (4-ounce) lobster tails

¼ cup extra-virgin olive oil

1 large clove garlic, minced

1 (28-ounce) can whole tomatoes

¼ teaspoon kosher salt

¼ teaspoon freshly ground black pepper

¼ teaspoon crushed red pepper flakes

5 large basil leaves

1 cup cooked brown rice

Phase I: Detox
Gluten Free (with gluten-free pasta)
Dairy Free
Egg Free

Serves 6
Serving size: ½ cup lobster,
½ cup rice
Yield: 3 cups lobster,
3 cups rice
Prep time: 10 minutes
Cook time: 30 minutes

Bring a medium pot of water to a boil. Add the lobster tails and cook for about 5 minutes, until the meat is firm. Remove the lobster and cool. When cool enough to handle, remove the lobster meat from the shells. Reserve both the meat and shells.

Heat the extra-virgin olive oil in a medium pot. Add the garlic and cook until just turning golden. Add the reserved lobster shells and cook briefly in the oil, for 1 to

2 minutes. Add the tomatoes, crushing them with your hands as you add them to the pot. Add the salt, pepper, and red pepper flakes. Bring to a simmer and cook for about 20 minutes, until the sauce is thickened. Remove the shells. Add the reserved lobster meat and the basil leaves.

Serve the lobster sauce over the cooked rice.

Nutritional Analysis

Per 1-cup serving: 444 Calories, 11 g Fat, 1.7 g Sat, 46 mg Chol,

10 g Fiber, 26 g Protein, 62 g Carb, 463 mg Sodium

Scallops Poached in Thai Coconut Curry Broth

This delicious preparation of scallops hits all flavor notes—salty, sweet, sour, and spicy. The coconut milk makes a smooth, but not too heavy, broth. The flavors of the ginger, lemongrass, and lime enhance the coconut broth. Coconut juice is easy to find in Asian and Latino markets. If unavailable, substitute filtered water. A tasty side dish with this curry is Mint-Scented Salad with Lime-Rice Wine Vinaigrette (page 86).

Phase I: Detox
Gluten Free
Dairy Free
Egg Free

Serves 4
Serving size: 6 ounces scallops plus 1 cup broth
Yield: 1½ pounds scallops plus 4 cups broth
Prep time: 15 minutes
Cook time: 55 minutes

2 cups organic low-sodium chicken stock or broth

2 (15-ounce) cans unsweetened lite coconut milk

1 cup coconut juice

½ cup sliced onion (about ½ small onion)

1 medium clove garlic, sliced

1 teaspoon Thai Kitchen Red Chili Paste

2 generous tablespoons peeled, sliced fresh ginger

1 large stalk of lemongrass, tough outside layer removed, thinly sliced

1 teaspoon finely grated lime zest

2 teaspoons fresh lime juice

1½ pounds sea scallops

2 cups cooked brown basmati rice

In a large saucepan, combine the chicken stock or broth, coconut milk, coconut juice, onion, garlic, and red chili paste. Bring to a simmer and cook over medium-low heat for 30 minutes.

Add the ginger and lemongrass and simmer for 20 minutes, until reduced to approximately 4 cups. Strain the broth and discard the solids. Add the lime zest and lime juice.

Heat the broth to a simmer and add the scallops. Cook for about 2 minutes, until just opaque in the center. Cook time will vary depending on the size of the scallops.

Serve the scallops and broth in bowls on a bed of brown basmati rice.

Nutritional Analysis

Per 6-ounces scallops plus 1 cup broth: 420 Calories, 15 g Fat, 12.3 g Sat,

69 mg Chol, 4 g Fiber, 38 g Protein, 37 g Carb, 450 mg Sodium

Grilled Lamb Chops with Garlic and Herbs

Phase I: Detox
Gluten Free
Dairy Free
Egg Free

Serves 4
Serving size: 2 (4-ounce)
chops
Yield: 8 chops
Prep time: 15 minutes plus
2 to 4 hours marinating
time
Cook time: 10 minutes

In this simple method of preparation, the herb-filled marinade enhances the flavor of the lamb. If desired, the lamb chops can be broiled indoors instead of grilled.

8 (1½-inch-thick) lamb loin chops (about 4 ounces each)

6 tablespoons extra-virgin olive oil

¼ cup low-sodium wheat-free tamari

2 tablespoons fresh lemon juice

2 large cloves garlic, chopped

3 tablespoons finely minced rosemary

1 tablespoons minced thyme leaves

1 tablespoons minced mint

1 teaspoon kosher salt

1 teaspoon freshly ground black pepper

Place the lamb chops in a single layer in a shallow baking dish.

Mix together the extra-virgin olive oil, tamari, lemon juice, garlic, rosemary, thyme, mint, salt, and pepper. Pour the marinade over the lamb chops, turning the chops to coat them thoroughly. Cover and refrigerate for 2 to 4 hours, turning lamb in the marinade every hour.

Preheat the grill to medium–high.

Wipe excess marinade off the lamb chops. Grill the chops for 6 minutes. Turn and continue grilling for 4 more minutes for medium-rare, or until desired degree of doneness is reached.

Nutritional Analysis

Per 2 (4-ounce) chop serving: 510 Calories, 30 g Fat, 8.2 g Sat, 182 mg Chol,

0 g Fiber, 58 g Protein, 0 g Carb, 480 mg Sodium

Herbed Rack of Lamb with Roasted Garlic and Shallots

This elegant, special-occasion entrée is quick and easy to prepare; just allow enough time to marinate the meat. The tiny chops are flavorful with herbs and garlic, tender and juicy when cooked to just pink in the center. For a colorful presentation, garnish with watercress.

Phase I: Detox
Gluten Free
Dairy Free
Egg Free

Serves 4
Serving size: 4 (1-ounce) chops
Yield: 16 chops
Prep time: 10 minutes plus 1 hour marinating time
Cook time: 20 minutes

2 (1- to 1¼-pound) racks of lamb, trimmed and frenched (about 8 ribs each)

1 tablespoon minced garlic (about 3 medium cloves)

1 tablespoon minced mint leaves

1 tablespoon minced parsley

1 tablespoon minced rosemary

1 teaspoon minced thyme

½ teaspoon kosher salt

½ teaspoon freshly ground black pepper

3 tablespoons extra-virgin olive oil

2 cups watercress, tough stems removed, for garnish

Place the lamb in a shallow dish. Combine the garlic, mint, parsley, rosemary, thyme, salt, pepper, and 2 tablespoons of extra-virgin olive oil. Spread evenly over the meaty surface of the lamb. Let stand at room temperature for up to 1 hour. If marinating for longer than 1 hour, place the rack of lamb in the refrigerator.

Preheat the oven to 425 degrees F.

Heat the remaining 1 tablespoon of extra-virgin olive oil in a large ovenproof skillet over medium-high heat. Add the lamb, meat side down. Sear for 2 minutes until brown. Turn the lamb rack over so that the meaty surface is facing up. Place the skillet in the oven and cook for about 18 minutes for medium rare, or until a meat thermometer inserted into the center reads about 125 degrees F. Let the lamb rest for about 10 to 15 minutes before carving. The internal temperature will rise to about 130 degrees F.

Slice the lamb into single or double chops, depending on your preference. Serve with Roasted Garlic and Shallots.

Nutritional Analysis

Per 4-chop serving: 446 Calories, 31 g Fat, 6.6 g Sat, 70 mg Chol,

0 g Fiber, 24 g Protein, 18 g Carb, 328 mg Sodium

Middle Eastern Lamb Patties

Phase I: Detox
Gluten Free
Dairy Free
Quick
Egg Free

Serves 6
Serving size: 1 (5-ounce)
lamb patty
Yield: 6 patties
Prep time: 20 minutes
Cook time: 10 to 12
minutes

Tasty and full of fresh herbs and warming spices, these patties are delicious grilled. Serve with a side of Mediterranean Chopped Salad (page 90). If Aleppo pepper is not available, use freshly ground black pepper.

2 pounds lean ground lamb

½ cup minced scallions (about 3 medium scallions)

⅓ cup minced red bell pepper (about ½ medium pepper)

¼ cup minced parsley

2 tablespoons minced cilantro

2 teaspoons Aleppo pepper

2 teaspoons minced garlic

1 teaspoon kosher salt

1 teaspoon ground coriander

½ teaspoon paprika

½ teaspoon ground cumin

2 teaspoons extra-virgin olive oil, for grilling

Place all ingredients, except the olive oil, in a medium bowl and gently combine the mixture, using care not to excessively compact the meat. Form into 6 patties, each about 1 inch thick.

Preheat an outdoor grill or a grill pan that has been brushed with the extra-virgin olive oil. Grill the lamb for about 5 to 6 minutes on each side for medium rare, or until desired degree of doneness.

Nutritional Analysis

Per 1 (5-ounce) patty: 244 Calories, 14 g Fat, 5.9 g Sat, 91 mg Chol,

1 g Fiber, 27 g Protein, 2 g Carb, 415 mg Sodium

Grilled Ginger Herbed Chicken Breasts

The herb marinade is subtle and forms a nice crust on the chicken breast when grilled. A splash of lime juice finishes the dish.

Phase I: Detox
Gluten Free
Dairy Free
Egg Free

Serves 4
Serving size: 1 (4-ounce)
chicken breast
Yield: 4 (4-ounce) chicken
breasts
Prep time: 20 minutes plus
1 hour marinating time
Cook time: 10 minutes

4 (about 1½ pounds total) boneless, skinless chicken breasts

¼ cup fresh lime juice

¼ cup extra-virgin olive oil

1 tablespoon minced fresh ginger

1 tablespoon minced oregano

2 teaspoons minced rosemary

2 medium cloves garlic, finely minced

½ teaspoon kosher salt

½ teaspoon red pepper flakes

½ teaspoon freshly ground black pepper

Lime wedges

Place the chicken breasts in a shallow baking dish.

Whisk together the lime juice, extra-virgin olive oil, ginger, oregano, rosemary, garlic, salt, and red and black pepper. Pour over the chicken. Cover and refrigerate for about 1 hour. Do not let sit for more than 2 hours, as this affects the texture of the chicken.

Preheat an outdoor grill, or a grill pan that has been brushed with extra-virgin olive oil, to medium-high. Grill the chicken for about 4 to 5 minutes on each side, or until juices run clear. Cooking time will vary with the thickness of the chicken.

Serve with lime wedges.

Nutritional Analysis

Per 4-ounce chicken breast: 203 Calories, 6 g Fat, 1.4 g Sat, 94 mg Chol,

0 g Fiber, 34 g Protein, 0 g Carb, 202 mg Sodium

Herbed Chicken Breasts

The secret to juicy chicken breasts is to not overcook. Pound the chicken breasts to an even ¼-inch thickness to cook quickly.

6 (about 2 pounds total) boneless, skinless chicken breast halves,
    pounded to ¼-inch thickness
3 tablespoons extra-virgin olive oil
2 teaspoons minced rosemary
2 teaspoons minced thyme
2 teaspoons minced oregano
2 teaspoons minced garlic
½ teaspoon kosher salt
½ teaspoon freshly ground black pepper

Phase I: Detox
Gluten Free
Dairy Free
Egg Free

Serves 6
Serving size: 1 (5-ounce) chicken breast
Yield: 6 (5-ounce) chicken breasts
Prep time: 15 minutes plus 1 hour marinating time
Cook time: 4 to 5 minutes

Place the chicken breasts in a shallow baking dish. Combine 2 tablespoons of extra-virgin olive oil, the rosemary, thyme, oregano, garlic, salt, and pepper. Pour over the chicken. Cover and refrigerate for 1 hour.

Heat the remaining extra-virgin olive oil in a large skillet over medium-high heat. Cook the chicken, in batches if necessary, for 2 minutes on each side. Remove the cooked chicken to a platter and keep warm while cooking the remaining breasts.

Nutritional Analysis
Per 5-ounce chicken breast: 231 Calories, 9 g Fat, 1.5 g Sat, 88 mg Chol,
0 g Fiber, 35 g Protein, 1 g Carb, 258 mg Sodium

Simple Grilled Chicken Breasts

Phase I: Detox
Gluten Free
Dairy Free
Quick
Egg Free

Serves 4
Serving size: 1 (4-ounce)
chicken breast
Yield: 4 (4-ounce) chicken
breasts
Prep time: 5 minutes
Cook time: 8 to 10 minutes

Grilling is the simplest of preparations for chicken, and the results are so delicious! Very versatile, these chicken breasts go with just about anything. Serve the pieces whole or sliced on the bias.

4 (about 1½ pounds total) boneless, skinless chicken breast halves

2 tablespoons extra-virgin olive oil

½ teaspoon kosher salt

½ teaspoon freshly ground black pepper

Rub the chicken breasts with the extra-virgin olive oil, salt, and pepper.

Preheat an outdoor grill, or a grill pan that has been brushed with extra-virgin olive oil, to medium-high. Grill or sauté the chicken for about 4 to 5 minutes on each side, or until the juices run clear. Cooking time will vary with the thickness of the chicken.

Nutritional Analysis

Per 4-ounce chicken breast: 245 Calories, 11 g Fat, 2.1 g Sat, 94 mg Chol,

0 g Fiber, 34 g Protein, 0 g Carb, 240 mg Sodium

Turkey and Red Bean Chili

Phase I: Detox
Gluten Free
Dairy Free
Egg Free

Serves 8
Serving size: 1 cup
Yield: 8 cups
Prep time: 25 minutes
Cook time: 1 hour to 1
hour and 10 minutes

Topped with cilantro and red onion, this ancho chile pepper–flavored turkey chili is spicy and flavorful.

⅓ cup extra-virgin olive oil

1 large onion, cut into ½-inch dice (about 1½ cups)

2 large cloves garlic, minced (about 1 tablespoon)

1 medium jalapeño pepper, seeded and minced (about 1 tablespoon)

2 pounds ground turkey breast

1 teaspoon kosher salt

1 (28-ounce) can low-sodium whole tomatoes

½ cup water

3 tablespoons ancho chile powder

4 teaspoons ground cumin

1½ teaspoons ground coriander

½ teaspoon freshly ground black pepper

¼ teaspoon hot paprika

2 tablespoons minced oregano

1 (15-ounce) can red beans, drained and rinsed

Chopped cilantro (optional)

Chopped red or green onion (optional)

8 (8-inch) sprouted corn tortillas

Heat the extra-virgin olive oil in a large, heavy-bottomed pan over medium heat. Add the onions and cook, stirring, for about 3 to 5 minutes, until translucent. Add the garlic and jalapeño and cook 1 minute longer.

Stir in the ground turkey and the salt and cook the turkey for about 5 minutes, breaking up the pieces with a wooden spoon, until it loses its pink color.

Crush the tomatoes with your hands and add them to the pan with their juice. Add the water and the ancho chile powder, cumin, coriander, black pepper, and paprika. Cook for 30 minutes at a gentle simmer, stirring occasionally.

Add the oregano and red beans and simmer for about 20 to 30 minutes, until the beans are heated through. Thin out the chili as desired with additional water if necessary.

Garnish as desired, just before serving, with one of the optional toppings, and serve with warm sprouted corn tortillas, wrapped in foil and heated in the oven at 300 degrees F. for about 5 minutes.

Nutritional Analysis

Per 1-cup serving: 302 Calories, 16 g Fat, 3.3 g Sat, 65 mg Chol,

4 g Fiber, 26 g Protein, 14 g Carb, 453 mg Sodium

Chicken Cacciatore

Phase I: Detox
Gluten Free
Dairy Free
Egg Free

Serves 6
Prep time: 25 minutes
Cook time: 40 minutes

A beautiful color and heady aroma make this the perfect dinner for a cold evening.

6 (about 3 pounds total) bone-in chicken breast halves, skin removed

¾ teaspoon kosher salt

1 teaspoon freshly ground black pepper

¼ cup plus 2 teaspoons extra-virgin olive oil

2 cups sliced onion (about 3 medium onions)

2 teaspoons minced garlic (about 2 medium cloves)

4 medium red bell peppers, cored, seeded, and cut into ½-inch strips

¼ cup organic low-sodium chicken broth

1 (28-ounce) can whole tomatoes, drained and chopped

1 teaspoon minced oregano

½ teaspoon minced rosemary

¼ teaspoon crushed red pepper flakes

½ pound cremini mushrooms, cut into thick slices

2 tablespoons finely chopped parsley

Rub the chicken with ½ teaspoon of the salt and ½ teaspoon of the black pepper.

Heat ¼ cup of the extra-virgin olive oil in a large skillet over medium-high heat. Add the chicken breasts and cook for about 4 to 5 minutes on each side, until brown. Remove the chicken to a platter and set aside.

Add the sliced onions to the pan and cook for about 5 minutes, until softened. Add the garlic and red peppers and cook for about 5 minutes, until the peppers begin to soften. Remove the onion-and red pepper mixture to a plate.

Add the broth to the skillet and bring to a boil over high heat. Cook for 1 minute, scraping any brown bits off the bottom of the pan. Add the tomatoes, oregano, rosemary, and crushed red pepper flakes, reduce to a simmer, and cook for 2 to 3 minutes, until slightly thickened. Stir in the reserved onions and peppers. Add the chicken pieces and bring back to a simmer. Cover and cook for 10 to 15 minutes, or until the chicken is done.

Meanwhile, heat the remaining 2 teaspoons of extra-virgin olive oil in a small skillet over medium-high heat. Add the mushrooms, the remaining ¼ teaspoon salt, and the remaining ½ teaspoon of black pepper. Cook for about 8 minutes, until the mushrooms have browned.

When the chicken is done, add the mushrooms to the pan and heat through. Adjust the seasoning if necessary. Serve garnished with the parsley.

Nutritional Analysis

Per serving: 339 calories, 9 g Fat, 1.6 g Sat, 105 mg Chol, 4 g Fiber, 47 g Protein, 19 g Carb, 456 mg Sodium

Soy-Marinated Tofu with Asian Vegetable Salad

Tofu infused with a mélange of Asian flavors and ingredients. Serve with Asian Vegetable Salad (page 82) for an attractive presentation. Allow time to press and drain the tofu before cooking.

Phase I: Detox
Gluten Free
Dairy Free
Vegetarian
Egg Free

Serves 4
Serving size: 1 slice tofu
plus 1 cup salad
Yield: 4 slices tofu plus 4
cups salad
Prep time: 10 minutes plus
1 hour or more to press,
drain, and marinate
Cook time: 6 minutes

1 (14-ounce) package extra-firm tofu

2 tablespoons low-sodium wheat-free tamari

2 tablespoons rice wine vinegar

1 tablespoon dark sesame oil

½ teaspoon Thai Kitchen Red Chili Paste

2 tablespoons light sesame oil

1 recipe Asian Vegetable Salad (page 82)

Cut the tofu into 2 equal pieces. Slice each piece in half, horizontally, making a total of 4 slices. To press and drain the tofu, place the slices in a single layer, on a shallow dish or tray, with paper towels underneath and on top of the tofu. Place another dish or tray on top of the tofu and weight it down with several cans of food or a heavy skillet. Refrigerate for at least 30 minutes.

Meanwhile, combine the tamari, rice wine vinegar, dark sesame oil, and red chili paste in a small bowl.

After the tofu has drained, discard the excess liquid and pat the tofu dry with a paper towel. Place the tofu in a shallow dish and pour the soy sauce marinade over it. Refrigerate for at least 30 minutes. Marinating longer will give the tofu a more intense flavor.

Heat the light sesame oil over medium–high heat in a skillet large enough to hold the tofu in a single layer. Cook the tofu for about 3 minutes on each side, until brown and beginning to crisp. Remove to a plate when finished cooking.

Serve with Asian Vegetable Salad.

Nutritional Analysis

Per 1 piece tofu and 1 cup salad: 292 Calories, 25 g Fat, 3.6 g Sat, 0 mg Chol,

2 g Fiber, 9 g Protein, 11 g Carb, 560 mg Sodium

Vegetable Tofu Scramble

This hearty, gluten-free vegetarian entrée also makes a nice breakfast. The tofu absorbs the flavor of the vegetables as it browns on the outside.

Phase I: Detox
Gluten Free
Dairy Free
Vegetarian
Egg Free

Serves 4
Serving size: 1 cup
Yield: 4 cups
Prep time: 25 minutes
Cook time: 12 minutes

1 (14-ounce) package firm tofu

2 tablespoons extra-virgin olive oil

¼ cup finely chopped shallots

½ cup diced red bell pepper (about ½ medium pepper)

1 cup roughly chopped shiitake mushrooms (about 6 medium mushrooms)

½ cup diced tomato

½ teaspoon minced garlic

¾ teaspoon kosher salt

½ teaspoon freshly ground black pepper

2 teaspoons minced oregano

12 chives, snipped into small pieces

Cut the tofu into 2 equal pieces. Slice each piece in half, horizontally, making a total of 4 slices. To press and drain the tofu, place the slices in a single layer, on a shallow dish or tray, with paper towels underneath and on top of the tofu. Place another dish or tray on top the tofu and weight it down with several cans of food or a heavy skillet. Refrigerate for at least 15 to 20 minutes. Cut the tofu into small cubes.

Heat the extra-virgin olive oil in a large skillet over medium heat. Add the shallots and red pepper and cook, stirring, for 3 minutes. Stir in the mushrooms, tomato, garlic, ½ teaspoon of the salt, and the pepper. Cook for 3 minutes. Increase the heat to medium-high and stir in the tofu, oregano, and remaining ¼ teaspoon salt.

Cook for 4 to 5 minutes, until the tofu has browned. Transfer to a plate and sprinkle with the chives.

Nutritional Analysis

Per 1-cup serving: 197 Calories, 15 g Fat, 2.3 g Sat, 0 mg Chol,

2 g Fiber, 14 g Protein, 6 g Carb, 376 mg Sodium

Avocado and Bean Burrito

Phase I: Detox
Gluten Free
Dairy Free
Quick
Vegetarian
Egg Free

Serves 2
Serving size: 1 burrito
Yield: 2 burritos
Prep time: 15 minutes
Cook time: none

A delicious, quick lunch.

2 cups shredded romaine lettuce

2 tablespoons yellow onion, chopped

½ medium avocado, peeled, pitted, and chopped

2 tablespoons chopped cilantro

4 tablespoons chunky tomato salsa

½ cup nonfat vegetarian refried beans

2 sprouted corn tortillas

Mix the lettuce, onion, avocado, cilantro, and salsa in a medium bowl until the vegetables are evenly coated. Smear half of the beans on each tortilla, fill with vegetable mixture, and wrap burrito style.

Nutritional Analysis

Per burrito: 288 Calories, 15 g Fat, 3.2 g Sat, 0 mg Chol, 9 g Fiber, 7 g Protein, 35 g Carb, 379 mg Sodium

Nutted Wild and Brown Rice Pilaf

This rustic-looking pilaf has a nice combination of colors from the carrot and parsley. The toasted hazelnuts add texture and a unique flavor.

Phase I: Detox
Gluten Free
Dairy Free
Vegetarian (with vegetable stock or broth)
Egg Free

Serves 8
Serving size: ½ cup
Yield: 4 cups
Prep time: 20 minutes
Cook time: 50 minutes

3 cups water

1 teaspoon kosher salt

¾ cup wild rice

2 tablespoons extra-virgin olive oil

½ cup finely chopped leek (about 1 small leek)

¼ cup finely chopped celery

¼ cup finely chopped carrot

1 teaspoon minced garlic (about 1 medium clove)

¾ cup brown rice

1½ cups organic low-sodium chicken or vegetable stock or broth

½ cup hazelnuts (about 2½ ounces)

2 tablespoons chopped parsley

½ teaspoon freshly ground black pepper

Bring the water to a boil and add ½ teaspoon of the salt. Add the wild rice and simmer for approximately 45 minutes, until tender yet firm. Drain and set aside.

Meanwhile, heat the extra-virgin olive oil in a large saucepan over medium heat. Add the leek, celery, and carrot. Cook, stirring, for 2 to 3 minutes, until just softened. Add the garlic and cook for 1 minute until fragrant, but not browned. Stir in the brown rice, coating the rice with the olive oil. Add the stock or broth and the remaining ½ teaspoon salt. Bring to a simmer, cover, and cook for about 35 to 40 minutes, until the broth is absorbed.

Meanwhile, toast the hazelnuts in a small skillet over medium heat for about 10 minutes. Stir the hazelnuts frequently and watch closely to prevent burning. When toasted, remove them from the pan and spread on a dish towel. Rub the nuts in the towel to remove the skins. Coarsely chop the nuts.

When the brown rice has cooked, stir in the cooked wild rice with a fork, fluffing the rice as it is mixed. Add the chopped toasted hazelnuts, parsley, and black pepper. Taste and adjust seasoning as needed.

Nutritional Analysis

Per ½-cup serving: 216 Calories, 10 g Fat, 1.1 g Sat, 1 mg Chol,

3 g Fiber, 6 g Protein, 28 g Carb, 216 mg Sodium

Coconut Dal with Steamed Broccoli and Brown Rice

Phase I: Detox
Gluten Free
Dairy Free
Vegetarian
Egg Free

Serves 6
Prep time: 10 minutes
Cook time: 30 minutes

This recipe can easily be doubled and frozen for later use as a convenient lunch or dinner.

2 cups yellow split peas

One 14-ounce can lite unsweetened coconut milk

4 cups low-sodium organic vegetable broth

1 small yellow onion, sliced

3 cloves garlic, pressed

1 tablespoon grated fresh ginger

2 teaspoons ground turmeric

1 teaspoon kosher salt

4 tablespoons chopped fresh cilantro

1 medium bunch broccoli, trimmed and steamed

1½ cups raw steamed brown rice

Rinse the split peas. In a large saucepan, place the split peas, coconut milk, vegetable broth, onion, garlic, ginger, turmeric, and salt. Simmer over medium heat until peas are soft, approximately 30 minutes. Sprinkle chopped fresh cilantro on top.

Serve with steamed broccoli and brown rice.

Nutritional Analysis

Per 1-cup serving dal and ½ cup rice: 427 Calories, 7 g Fat, 5.3 g Sat, 0 mg Chol,

20 g Fiber, 20 g Protein, 54 g Carb, 491 mg Sodium

Per 1-cup serving broccoli: 60 Calories, 0 g Fat, 0 g Sat, 0 mg Chol,

6 g Fiber, 4 g Protein, 12 g Carb, 32 mg Sodium

Braised Kale with Mushrooms and Beans

Great Northern beans or navy beans are best in this hearty vegetable side dish or vegetarian main course. Mix mushrooms such as shiitake, cremini, and white button.

Phase I: Detox
Gluten Free
Dairy Free
Vegetarian (with vegetable broth)
Egg Free

Serves 6
Serving size: ⅔ cup
Yield: 4 cups
Prep time: 30 minutes
Cook time: 40 minutes

2 tablespoons extra-virgin olive oil

⅓ cup minced shallot

1 teaspoon minced garlic

½ pound mixed mushrooms, stems removed, sliced

½ teaspoon kosher salt

1 medium bunch of kale (about 1 to 1¼ pounds), tough stems removed,
   cut into 1-inch strips

½ cup organic low-sodium chicken or vegetable broth

1 cup canned low-sodium or cooked white beans, such as navy or Great Northern,
   drained and rinsed

¼ teaspoon freshly ground black pepper

Heat 1 tablespoon of the extra-virgin olive oil in a large skillet over medium–high heat. Add half of the shallot and cook for about 5 minutes, until translucent. Add half of the garlic and cook, stirring, for 1 to 2 minutes.

Add the mushrooms and ¼ teaspoon of the salt. Cook the mushrooms for about 6 minutes, until they have released their liquid and have begun to brown. Remove the mushrooms from the pan and set aside.

Heat the remaining 1 tablespoon of extra-virgin olive oil in the skillet over medium–high heat. Add the remaining shallot and cook for about 5 minutes, until translucent. Add the remaining garlic and cook, stirring, for 1 to 2 minutes.

Add the sliced kale, broth, remaining ¼ teaspoon salt, and a pinch of pepper. Turn the kale in the pan until it wilts. Cover the pan and cook, stirring occasionally, for about 25 minutes, until the kale is tender.

Add the white beans, cooked mushrooms, and black pepper. Heat through and serve.

Nutritional Analysis

Per ⅔-cup serving: 119 Calories, 5.4 g Fat, 0.8 g Sat, 0 mg Chol,

3 g Fiber, 5 g Protein, 13 g Carb, 208 mg Sodium

Crabmeat Salad with Avocado and Mango

Here an extra-virgin olive oil and lime-based dressing stands in for the oft-used mayonnaise in this pretty, colorful salad with a great combination of taste and texture.

Phase I: Detox
Gluten Free
Dairy Free
Quick
Egg Free

Serves 8
Serving size: ½ cup
Yield: 4 cups
Prep time: 25 minutes
Cook time: none

1 pound lump crabmeat, picked over to remove any shells

¼ cup minced scallion

¼ cup diced fennel

¼ cup finely diced red bell pepper

¼ cup minced cilantro

1 teaspoon minced jalapeño pepper

1 teaspoon lime zest

5 tablespoons extra-virgin olive oil

4 tablespoons fresh lime juice

½ teaspoon kosher salt

½ teaspoon freshly ground black pepper

2 avocados, halved, pitted, peeled, and each half cut into 8 thin slices

1 cup diced mango

2 tablespoons snipped chives

Flake the crabmeat into a bowl. Gently fold in the scallion, fennel, red pepper, cilantro, jalapeño pepper, and lime zest.

Combine 4 tablespoons of the extra-virgin olive oil, 3 tablespoons of the lime juice, and the salt and pepper. Pour over the crab and gently mix.

Combine the remaining 1 tablespoon extra-virgin olive oil and 1 tablespoon lime juice with a pinch of salt. Fan 4 avocado slices on each plate. Drizzle with the extra-virgin olive oil and lime juice mixture. Place the crab salad at the base of the avocado on the plate. Place 2 tablespoons of the mango on one side of the crab. Sprinkle with the chives.

Nutritional Analysis

Per ½-cup serving: 228 Calories, 17 g Fat, 2.3 g Sat, 57 mg Chol, 4 g Fiber, 13 g Protein, 9 g Carb, 284 mg Sodium

Lentil Salad

French green lentils are preferable, as they remain firm after cooking and create a beautiful salad. Serve the lentils warm or at room temperature.

Phase I: Detox
Gluten Free
Dairy Free
Vegetarian
Egg Free

Serves 6
Serving size: ½ cup
Yield: about 3 cups
Prep time: 20 minutes
Cook time: 40 minutes

1 cup French green lentils

1 bay leaf

1 clove garlic, peeled

¼ small onion

1 rib celery with leaves, cut in half

½ teaspoon kosher salt

¼ cup finely chopped carrot

¼ cup minced parsley

¼ cup finely chopped fennel

2 tablespoons minced red onion

2 teaspoons minced oregano

1 teaspoon minced garlic

¼ cup extra-virgin olive oil

2 tablespoons fresh lemon juice

½ teaspoon freshly ground black pepper

Place the lentils, bay leaf, garlic, onion, and celery in a medium saucepan. Bring to a simmer and cook for about 30 minutes, until lentils are cooked but still slightly firm. Add ¼ teaspoon of the salt and continue cooking for about 10 minutes, until the lentils are tender. Drain the lentils, discarding the bay leaf, garlic clove, and celery. Transfer the lentils to a bowl. Stir in the carrot, parsley, fennel, red onion, oregano, and minced garlic.

Whisk together the extra-virgin olive oil, lemon juice, the remaining ¼ teaspoon salt, and the pepper and pour over the salad. Mix well.

Nutritional Analysis

Per ½-cup serving: 190 Calories, 10 g Fat, 1.3 g Sat, 0 mg Chol, 5 g Fiber, 7 g Protein, 19 g Carb, 170 mg Sodium

Seafood Salad with Lemon Dressing

Phase I: Detox
Gluten Free
Dairy Free
Egg Free

Serves 8
Serving size: 1 cup
Yield: 8 cups
Prep time: 30 minutes
Cook time: 1½ hours

While this may take a little more time to prepare than the average green salad, the results are well worth the effort. The selection of seafood can vary according to taste. No matter what the seafood selection, this is a beautiful first course, luncheon entrée, or al fresco dinner entrée, especially alfresco on a warm summer night.

18 littleneck clams, soaked in water and drained to remove sand

1 pound small mussels (about 2 dozen), scrubbed, black "beard" removed, and soaked in cold water

1 teaspoon kosher salt

6 black peppercorns

1 bay leaf

1 pound large (21 to 25 count) shrimp, peeled and deveined

1 pound sea scallops, rinsed

2 pounds whole squid, cleaned, cut into ¼-inch rings, and large tentacles cut in half

1 large rib celery, chopped

10 pitted Kalamata olives, chopped

5 pitted green Sicilian olives, chopped

1 medium red pepper, roasted (page 150), peeled, and chopped

¼ cup fresh lemon juice

1 medium clove garlic, minced

1 tablespoon minced oregano

½ teaspoon freshly ground black pepper

¾ cup extra-virgin olive oil

Discard any clams or mussels that are cracked, opened, or do not close when tapped with your finger.

Put 2 quarts of water in a large pot. Add the salt, peppercorns, and bay leaf. Bring the water to a boil and add the shrimp. Cook for 2 to 3 minutes, until the shrimp are pink and cooked throughout. Remove the shrimp with a slotted spoon and place in a large bowl.

Bring the water back to a boil and add the scallops. Cook for about 2 minutes, until the scallops just turn opaque. When cooked, remove to the bowl with the shrimp.

Return the water to a boil and add the squid. Bring to a boil and cook for about 1 minute. When cooked, remove to the bowl with the shrimp and scallops.

Put the clams in a separate saucepan with ¼ cup of water. Cover and cook over medium-high heat until the shells open. Discard any clams that do not open. Remove the clams, leaving the water in the pan. When cool enough to handle, remove the cooked clams from the shells and add to the bowl with the other shellfish.

Put the mussels in the same pan that was used for the clams. Cover and cook over medium-high heat until the shells open. Discard any that do not open. Remove the mussels from the pan. When cool enough to handle, remove the mussels from the shells and add to the bowl with the other shellfish.

Stir the chopped celery, olives, and roasted red pepper into the seafood.

Whisk together the lemon juice, garlic, oregano, and pepper. Slowly whisk in the extra-virgin olive oil until the dressing is slightly thickened. Pour about two-thirds of the dressing on the salad and mix gently. Let the salad stand for about 2 hours at room temperature.

Taste the salad, and if necessary add more dressing and pepper as desired.

Nutritional Analysis

Per 1-cup serving: 485 Calories, 27 g Fat, 4.0 g Sat, 416 mg Chol,

1 g Fiber, 49 g Protein, 10 g Carb, 259 mg Sodium

Southwestern Corn and Black Bean Salad

Flavorful and full of color, this salad has crunch from the onion and corn, with a soft texture from the black beans and diced avocado. The lime-flavored dressing adds spark, but for more heat, increase the minced jalapeño pepper. Garnish with the avocado just before serving.

Phase I: Detox
Gluten Free
Dairy Free
Quick
Vegetarian
Egg Free

Serves 6
Serving size: ½ cup
Yield: 3 cups
Prep time: 30 minutes
Cook time: none

1½ cups fresh or frozen corn kernels, thawed (about 3 ears fresh corn)

1 (15-ounce) can low-sodium black beans, drained and rinsed,
    or 1½ cups cooked black beans

½ cup diced roasted red pepper (page 150)

6 tablespoons finely diced red onion

¼ cup chopped cilantro, leaves and tender stems included

2 teaspoons minced jalapeño pepper

3 tablespoons fresh lime juice

½ teaspoon kosher salt

½ teaspoon ground cumin

¼ teaspoon freshly ground black pepper

⅛ teaspoon ground red pepper

3 tablespoons extra-virgin olive oil

1 medium avocado, peeled, pitted, and diced (about 1 cup), for garnish

Mix together the corn, beans, red pepper, red onion, cilantro, and jalapeño pepper.

Whisk together the lime juice, salt, cumin, black pepper, and ground red pepper. Slowly whisk in the extra-virgin olive oil until the dressing is slightly thickened.

Pour the dressing over the beans and stir to combine. Let the salad stand for about 1 hour to develop the flavors.

Prepare the avocado, and either gently fold it into the salad or garnish with the avocado immediately before serving.

Nutritional Analysis

Per ½-cup serving: 156 Calories, 8 g Fat, 1.1 g Sat, 0 mg Chol, 4 g Fiber, 5 g Protein, 19 g Carb, 181 mg Sodium

White Bean Salad with Roasted Red Pepper and Fennel

A beautiful main-course salad, perfect for lunch, the creamy white beans are complemented by crunchy fennel and the smoky taste of the roasted red pepper. Fresh scallion and parsley add bright green color and flavor to the other ingredients.

Phase I: Detox
Gluten Free
Dairy Free
Quick
Vegetarian
Egg Free

Serves 4
Serving size: ½ cup
Yield: 2 cups
Prep time: 20 minutes
Cook time: none

.1 (15-ounce) can low-sodium or 2 cups cooked Great Northern beans, drained and rinsed

1 cup diced roasted red pepper (page 150)

½ cup diced fennel

10 to 12 leaves fresh basil, cut into slivers (about ¼ cup)

2 tablespoons minced scallion (about 1 large scallion)

2 tablespoons finely chopped parsley

¼ cup extra-virgin olive oil

2 tablespoons fresh lemon juice

½ teaspoon finely minced garlic (about 1 small clove)

½ teaspoon kosher salt

½ teaspoon freshly ground black pepper

Mix together the beans, roasted pepper, fennel, basil, scallion, and parsley in a medium bowl.

Whisk together the extra-virgin olive oil, lemon juice, minced garlic, salt, and the black pepper in a small bowl. Pour the dressing over the beans.

Nutritional Analysis

Per ½-cup serving: 236 Calories, 14 g Fat, 2 g Sat, 0 mg Chol,

7 g Fiber, 6.5 g Protein, 42 g Carb, 261 mg Sodium

Parslied Lentil Salad

This is a great salad to make ahead of time for a "grab and go" lunch and it stores well in the refrigerator for a few days.

Phase I: Detox
Gluten Free
Dairy Free
Quick
Egg Free

Serves 4
Serving size: 1 cup
Yield: 4 cups
Prep time: 20 minutes
Cook time: none

6 tablespoons freshly squeezed lemon juice

⅓ cup extra-virgin olive oil

1 15-ounce can low-sodium lentils, drained

1 small chopped red onion

1 cup grated carrots

1 cup chopped fresh parsley

1 cup chopped green olives

In a large bowl, whisk together the lemon juice and olive oil. Add the lentils, onion, carrots, parsley, and green olives and toss to blend. Refrigerate for a few hours so that flavors can meld.

Nutritional Analysis

Per 1-cup serving: 347 Calories, 22 g Fat, 3 g Sat, 0 mg Chol,

11 g Fiber, 10 g Protein, 32 g Carb, 322 mg Sodium

Pasta Pesto Salad

Pesto and pasta are a delicious and filling combination that you can enjoy as long as you are conscientious about the ingredients you use. Make sure to use a bean flour pasta for this dish to keep your intake of white flour low. Pesto Sauce can be stored in the refrigerator for a few days.

Phase I: Detox
Gluten Free
Dairy Free
Quick
Vegetarian
Egg Free

Serves 2
Serving size: 2 cups
Yield: 4 cups
Prep time: 20 minutes
Cook time: 15 minutes

Pesto Sauce

⅓ cup pine nuts

2 cups fresh basil leaves, washed and stems removed

3 cloves garlic, pressed

2 tablespoons extra-virgin olive oil

4 tablespoons freshly squeezed lemon juice

dash kosher salt

pinch freshly ground black pepper

Pesto Salad

1 cup broccoli florets

1 cup cauliflower florets

1 chopped red bell pepper

1 sliced carrot

4 ounces dry bean flour pasta

Cook pasta according to package directions until al dente. While pasta is cooking, mix the pine nuts, basil, garlic, olive oil, lemon juice, salt and pepper in a small food processor and puree until smooth. Place vegetables in a large mixing bowl and set aside. Drain pasta and pour hot pasta water over vegetables. Blanch vegetables in pasta water for 3 minutes. Drain blanched vegetables, add cooked pasta and approximately 2 tablespoons of the pesto sauce and toss gently until mixed. Refrigerate for 2–3 hours for flavors to marinate.

Nutritional Analysis

Per 2-cup serving: 100 Calories, 10 g Fat, 3.7 g Sat, 0 mg Chol, 1 g Fiber, 2 g Protein, 3g Carb, 1 mg Sodium

Pasta Salad: 258 Calories, 1 g Fat, 0 g Sat, 0 mg Chol, 12 g Fiber, 22 g Protein, 56 g Carb, 57 mg Sodium

Totals: 358 Calories, 11 g Fat, 3.7 g Sat, 0 mg Chol, 13 g Fiber, 24 g Protein, 59 g Carb, 58 mg Sodium

Cajun Black-Eyed Peas

Phase I: Detox
Gluten Free
Dairy Free
Quick
Vegetarian
Egg Free

Serves 4
Serving size: 2 cups
Yield: 8 cups
Prep time: 15 minutes
Cook time: 30 minutes

Traditionally black-eyed peas are cooked on New Year's Day for good luck. This version adds cayenne pepper to create a nice spicy flavor. Cayenne is also a detoxifying spice, so you get to take advantage of that as well. Serve this dish over brown rice for a hearty dinner or alone as a light lunch.

1 tablespoon extra-virgin olive oil

7 stalks green onions or scallions, chopped

⅓ cup diced red onion

2 cloves garlic, peeled and minced

4 teaspoons diced poblano pepper

¾ cup organic low-sodium vegetable broth

2 15-ounce cans black-eyed peas

1 tablespoon lemon juice

½ teaspoon cayenne pepper

⅛ teaspoon crushed red pepper flakes

½–1 teaspoon kosher salt

3 tablespoons chopped fresh cilantro

Heat olive oil in a large pot over medium heat until hot. Add all onions, garlic, and poblano pepper. Sauté the vegetables for 2–3 minutes until aromatic then add the vegetable broth.

Pour beans from can into strainer and rinse with cold water.

Add the beans, lemon juice, and all spices and herbs to the vegetable broth. Simmer 20–25 minutes while stirring occasionally until beans and vegetables are soft.

Remove from heat and either enjoy warm or chill and serve.

Nutritional Analysis

Per 2-cup serving: 178 Calories, 4 g Fat, 0 g Sat, 0 mg Chol, 7 g Fiber, 10 g Protein, 28 g Carb, 322 mg Sodium

Curried Vegetables with Coconut Milk

Curry is a delicious way to eat veggies along with the healthy saturated fat in coconut milk. It's good hot or cold.

Phase I: Detox
Gluten Free
Dairy Free
Quick
Vegetarian
Egg Free

Serves 4
Serving size: 1 cup
Yield: 4 cups
Prep time: 15 minutes
Cook time: 30 minutes

1 tablespoon extra-virgin olive oil

2 tablespoons diced poblano pepper

1 cup sliced red onion

1 clove garlic, peeled and minced

2 teaspoons fresh ginger

⅓ cup sliced carrots

⅓ cup diced celery

4 cups (½ head) 1½" pieces cauliflower

½ cup organic low-sodium vegetable broth

¼ teaspoon cumin

¼ teaspoon curry powder

¼ teaspoon cayenne pepper

½ teaspoon kosher salt

¼ cup lite coconut milk

1 tablespoon lemon juice

1 teaspoon fresh cilantro

Heat olive oil on medium heat in a sauté pan. Add the pepper, onion, garlic, ginger, carrots, and celery. Sauté vegetables until tender, about 8–10 minutes. Add the cauliflower, vegetable broth, and all the spices. Bring to a simmer (do not boil). Cover and cook an additional 10–15 minutes, stirring as needed.

Once the cauliflower is tender, stir in the coconut milk, lemon juice, and cilantro. Bring contents of pan back to a simmer for 3–5 minutes and allow liquid to thicken slightly.

Remove from heat.

Nutritional Analysis

Per 1-cup serving: 134 Calories, 9 g Fat, 3 g Sat, 0 mg Chol, 4 g Fiber, 3 g Protein, 12 g Carb, 338 mg Sodium

Quinoa and Garbanzo Bean Salad

Phase I: Detox
Gluten Free
Dairy Free
Quick
Vegetarian
Egg Free

Serves 4
Serving size: 1 cup
Yield: 4 cups
Prep time: 10 minutes
Cook time: 30 minutes

Light, refreshing, and delicious, this is a perfect vegetarian entree for a warm afternoon. It is best made ahead to let the flavors blend. The quinoa can also be cooked in a rice cooker.

1½ cups water

¾ cup quinoa

1 tablespoon extra-virgin olive oil

½ cup chopped onion

½ cup diced poblano pepper

¼ cup (3 scallions) sliced green onions or scallions

¾ cup chickpeas, canned

Dressing

2 tablespoons lemon juice

½ teaspoon chili powder

½ teaspoons fresh oregano

1 teaspoon fresh parsley

½ teaspoon kosher salt

2 tablespoons extra-virgin olive oil

Bring water to a boil. Add quinoa and stir. Turn down heat to low. Cover. Simmer covered 25–30 minutes, until all water is absorbed and quinoa is tender. Cool cooked quinoa.

Drain canned chick peas and rinse.

Heat oil in a medium skillet. Sauté onion and pepper over medium heat for 2–5 minutes or until onion is slightly soft.

In a large bowl, mix thoroughly onion-pepper mixture, green onions, cooked quinoa, and chick peas.

Dressing: In a small bowl, add lemon juice, chili powder, oregano, parsley, and salt. Slowly whisk in olive oil. Pour dressing over quinoa-chickpea mixture. Gently mix until dressing thoroughly covers all the salad.

Nutritional Analysis

Per 1-cup serving: 227 Calories, 9 g Fat, 1 g Sat, 0 mg Chol, 4 g Fiber, 6 g Protein, 31 g Carb, 47 mg Sodium

Three Bean Vegetarian Chili

We offer another vegetarian chili here that tastes best the day after its made. This one gives you the option of incorporating three different types of beans to increase your phytonutrient intake.

Phase I: Detox
Gluten Free
Dairy Free
Vegetarian
Egg Free

Serves 4
Serving size: 1½ cups
Yield: 6 cups
Prep time: 10 minutes
Cook time: 60 minutes

1 cup canned black eyed peas

⅔ cup canned chickpeas

½ cup canned Great Northern beans

1 tablespoon extra-virgin olive oil

¼ cup diced onion

1 clove garlic, peeled and minced

¼ cup diced celery

⅔ cup diced poblano pepper

2 cups organic low-sodium vegetable broth

1 tablespoon chili powder

¼ teaspoon chopped fresh parsley

¼ teaspoon cumin

¼ teaspoon fresh thyme

⅛ teaspoon cayenne pepper

¼ cup kosher salt

Drain and rinse beans

Heat oil in a stock pot over medium heat. Sauté onion, garlic, celery, and peppers for 5–7 minutes.

Add vegetable broth, beans, and parsley and spices. Cover. Simmer for approximately 1 hour or until beans are tender and liquid thickens slightly.

Remove from heat and chill.

Nutritional Analysis

Per 1½-cup serving: 112 Calories, 3 g Fat, 0 g Sat, 0 mg Chol, 4 g Fiber, 5 g Protein, 17 g Carb, 545 mg Sodium

Tuscan White Bean Stew

Phase I: Detox
Gluten Free
Dairy Free
Vegetarian
Egg Free

Serves 4
Serving size: 1½ cups
Yield: 6 cups
Prep time: 10 minutes
Cook time: 35 minutes

This stew has a delicate flavor. For a deeper flavor, try roasting the garlic. Serve warm or chilled.

1 15-ounce can organic great northern beans

1 tablespoon extra-virgin olive oil

¼ cup diced onion

½ cup diced carrots

⅓ cup diced celery

1 clove garlic, peeled and minced

2 cups organic low-sodium vegetable broth

⅛ teaspoon fresh rosemary

¼ teaspoon fresh parsley

¼ teaspoon fresh thyme

½ teaspoon kosher salt

Drain beans, rinse, and dry.

In a stock pot, heat oil over medium–low heat. Sauté onions for 2–3 minutes. Add carrots, celery, and garlic. Sauté for an additional 4–5 minutes or until vegetables start to become soft. Add vegetable broth, beans, and all herbs and salt. Simmer covered for 20–30 minutes, stirring occasionally.

Remove from heat and serve or chill for later.

Nutritional Analysis

Per 1½-cup serving: 106 Calories, 2 g Fat, 0 g Sat, 0 mg Chol, 4 g Fiber, 5 g Protein, 18 g Carb, 874 mg Sodium

Vegetable Curry with Chickpeas

Adding chickpeas to your curry thickens it and gives it a robust nutty flavor. Serve with brown rice for a hearty meal.

Phase I: Detox
Gluten Free
Dairy Free
Vegetarian
Egg Free

Serves 4
Serving size: 1 cup
Yield: 4 cups
Prep time: 25 minutes
Cook time: 35 minutes

1 tablespoon extra-virgin olive oil

1–2 tablespoons diced poblano pepper

1 cup diced white onion

1–2 cloves garlic, peeled and minced

2 tablespoons peeled and minced fresh ginger

⅓ cup ¼" slices carrot

⅓ cup diced celery

1½ cups 1½" pieces cauliflower

1 (15-ounce) can low-sodium chickpeas, rinsed and drained

¾ cup organic low-sodium vegetable broth

1 teaspoon curry powder

½ teaspoon cumin

⅛ teaspoon cayenne pepper

1½ teaspoon kosher salt

¼ cup lite coconut milk

1 tablespoon lemon juice

1 teaspoon chopped fresh cilantro

In a stock pot, heat olive oil over medium heat. Once the oil is hot add peppers, onions, garlic, ginger, carrots, and celery. Sauté vegetables until tender, about 8–10 minutes (cover pot as needed).

Add the cauliflower, chickpeas, vegetable broth, and all spices. Bring to a simmer (do not boil) for 20 minutes, stirring as needed. Once the cauliflower is tender, stir in the coconut milk, lemon juice, and cilantro. Bring pot back to a simmer for 3–5 minutes so the liquid can thicken slightly.

Remove from heat and eat warm or chill and eat later.

Nutritional Analysis

Per 1-cup serving: 209 Calories, 11 g Fat, 5 g Sat, 0 mg Chol, 6 g Fiber, 7 g Protein, 22 g Carb, 495 mg Sodium

Braised Carrots with Parsley and Chives

The carrots are cooked whole, making an interesting presentation. Simple to prepare, sweet in flavor, and beautiful to look at, serve this as a side dish for meat, poultry, or fish.

Phase I: Detox
Gluten Free
Dairy Free
Quick
Vegetarian
Egg Free

Serves 6
Serving size: 2 carrots
Yield: 12 carrots
Prep time: 10 minutes
Cook time: 10 minutes

2 bunches (about 12) whole carrots

2 tablespoons extra-virgin olive oil

½ teaspoon kosher salt

¼ teaspoon freshly ground black pepper

⅓ cup water

1 tablespoon chopped parsley

1 tablespoon snipped chives

1 teaspoon lemon zest

Remove the leaves from the carrots and peel the carrots.

Place the carrots in a large skillet over medium-high heat with the extra-virgin olive oil, salt, and pepper and cook, stirring, until the carrots begin to brown.

Add the water. Bring to a boil, reduce the heat to medium-high, and cook, covered, for about 10 minutes, until the carrots are tender and browned.

Remove from the heat and sprinkle with the chopped parsley, snipped chives, and lemon zest.

Nutritional Analysis

Per 2-carrot serving: 102 Calories, 5 g Fat, 0.7 g Sat, 0 mg Chol,

4 g Fiber, 1 g Protein, 14 g Carb, 260 mg Sodium

Chopped Broccoli with Olives

Phase I: Detox
Gluten Free
Dairy Free
Vegetarian
Egg Free

Serves 8
Serving size: ½ cup
Yield: 4 cups
Prep time: 20 minutes
Cook time: 15 minutes

Broccoli and olives are a beautiful combination. The garlic and lemon zest enhance the flavor.

1 medium head broccoli (about 1¼ pounds)

2 tablespoons extra-virgin olive oil

1 teaspoon minced garlic

Pinch of red pepper flakes

½ teaspoon kosher salt

¼ cup pitted chopped Kalamata olives

1 tablespoon minced parsley

¼ teaspoon lemon zest

Chop the broccoli into small florets. Peel the stems and cut into ½-inch pieces.

Bring a large pot of salted water to a boil. Drop in the broccoli florets and cook for 1 to 2 minutes, until crisp-tender. Transfer to a bowl of ice water to stop the cooking. Drain and set aside.

Heat the extra-virgin olive oil in a medium skillet over medium heat. Add the minced garlic and cook for about 1 minute, until the garlic is just beginning to color.

Add the broccoli, red pepper flakes, and salt and cook, stirring, for 2 to 3 minutes.

Add the olives, parsley, and lemon zest. Cook, stirring, until heated throughout.

Nutritional Analysis

Per ½ cup serving: 62 Calories, 5.5 g Fat, .75 g Sat, 0 mg Chol,

1 g Fiber, 1 g Protein, 2.5 g Carb, 245 mg Sodium

The UltraMetabolism Cookbook

Edamame and Grilled Corn Succotash

This recipe is best made with fresh, sweet summertime corn.

1 cup frozen shelled edamame

3 medium ears corn, silks and husks removed (about 1½ cups kernels)

½ cup chopped roasted red pepper (page 150)

¼ cup finely diced sweet onion, such as Vidalia

2 tablespoons fresh lime juice

1 teaspoon finely grated lemon zest

1 teaspoon minced garlic

½ teaspoon kosher salt

½ teaspoon freshly ground black pepper

2 tablespoons extra-virgin olive oil

¼ cup minced cilantro

Phase I: Detox
Gluten Free
Dairy Free
Quick
Vegetarian
Egg Free

Serves 6
Serving size: ½ cup
Yield: 3 cups
Prep time: 25 minutes
Cook time: 5 to 10 minutes

Bring a large pan of salted water to a boil. Drop in the edamame and cook for about 3 to 4 minutes, until tender yet firm. Drain and place in a bowl of ice water to stop the cooking. Drain and shake dry. Place in a medium bowl.

Grill the corn for about 3 minutes on a gas stove, directly over the gas flame. Alternatively, grill on an indoor or outdoor grill until slightly charred, about 3 minutes, turning the corn to grill evenly. Let cool, and cut the kernels off the cob.

Stir the corn into the edamame. Add the red pepper and onion.

Combine the lime juice, lemon zest, garlic, salt, and pepper. Slowly whisk in the extra-virgin olive oil until slightly thickened. Pour the dressing over the vegetables. Stir in the cilantro.

Nutritional Analysis

Per ½-cup serving: 122 Calories, 6 g Fat, 0.8 g Sat, 0 mg Chol, 2 g Fiber, 5 g Protein, 14 g Carb, 191 mg Sodium

Phase I: Detox
Gluten Free
Dairy Free
Quick
Vegetarian
Egg Free

Serves 4
Serving size: ½ cup
Yield: 2 cups
Prep time: 15 minutes
Cook time: 10 minutes

Fire-Roasted Red Peppers with Garlic and Capers

This recipe results in beautiful, shiny roasted red peppers bathed in olive oil and studded with garlic and capers. The peppers are delicious layered on sandwiches; they also make a wonderful addition to any antipasto platter or buffet table. The peppers can be roasted under the broiler, directly on a gas flame on the stovetop, or on an outdoor grill.

5 medium red peppers (about 1½ pounds)

4 tablespoons extra-virgin olive oil

2 tablespoons capers

1 medium clove garlic, pressed or finely chopped

¼ teaspoon kosher salt

¼ teaspoon freshly ground black pepper

Broiler method: Preheat the broiler to high. Lay the peppers on a sheet pan and place under the broiler 2 to 3 inches from the element. Cook, turning with tongs, until charred on all sides.

Stovetop method: Place the whole peppers directly on the gas flame, turning with tongs, until charred on all sides.

Outdoor grill method: Preheat the grill to high. Lay the whole peppers in the grill grate and cook, turning with tongs, until charred on all sides.

Place the charred peppers in a bowl and cover tightly with plastic wrap, or in a large saucepan with a tight-fitting lid. When the peppers are cool enough to handle, remove the charred skin, the core, and the seeds. The skin will come off easily. Do not run the peppers under water, as this will decrease their flavor. Peel over a plate and save any juices that drain from the peppers. Cut the pepper flesh into wide strips. Place a layer of the strips in a shallow dish and top with some of the

extra-virgin olive oil, capers, garlic, salt, and pepper. Repeat the layering with the remaining ingredients. Pour any accumulated juice over the assembled dish.

Nutritional Analysis

Per ½-cup serving: 168 Calories, 15 g Fat, 1.0 g Sat, 0 mg Chol, 3 g Fiber, 2 g Protein, 9 g Carb, 250 mg Sodium

Grilled Asparagus with Lemon Zest, Garlic, and Parsley

Grilled asparagus are best in the spring, when they are in season. This marvelous side dish is further enhanced with a sprinkle of fresh herbs, garlic, and citrus zest.

Phase I: Detox
Gluten Free
Dairy Free
Quick
Vegetarian
Egg Free

Serves 4
Serving size: ¼ pound
Yield: 1 pound
Prep time: 15 minutes
Cook time: 5 to 10 minutes

2 medium cloves garlic, minced (about 2 teaspoons)
2 teaspoons finely minced parsley
1 teaspoon grated lemon zest
2 tablespoons extra-virgin olive oil
1 pound asparagus, trimmed and tough stem ends removed
½ teaspoon kosher salt
½ teaspoon freshly ground black pepper

In a small bowl, combine the minced garlic, parsley, and lemon zest.

Brush a grill pan with 1 tablespoon of the extra-virgin olive oil and heat over medium-high heat.

Toss the asparagus with the remaining 1 tablespoon extra-virgin olive oil, the salt, and pepper. Grill for about 10 minutes, until golden brown but still crisp-tender. Cook time will vary with the thickness of the asparagus.

Transfer to a platter and sprinkle with the garlic, parsley, and lemon zest mixture.

Nutritional Analysis

Per ¼-pound serving: 79 Calories, 7.5 g Fat, 1.0 g Sat, 0 mg Chol, 1 g Fiber, 1 g Protein, 3 g Carb, 248 mg Sodium

Grilled Vegetables with Lemon and Mint

Phase I: Detox
Gluten Free
Dairy Free
Quick
Vegetarian
Egg Free

Serves 6
Prep time: 20 minutes
Cook time: 10 to 20
minutes

Best cooked on an outdoor grill and arranged on a platter, these vegetables are beautiful. Vary the vegetables—try asparagus, thick-sliced onions, large mushroom caps, or halved leeks—using this method to make many delicious combinations.

2 baby eggplants

2 red or yellow peppers, cored, seeded, and cut into 3-inch strips

2 small zucchini, ends removed and sliced diagonally into ¼-inch-thick slices

5 tablespoons extra-virgin olive oil

½ teaspoon kosher salt

½ teaspoon freshly ground black pepper

1 teaspoon minced garlic (1 medium clove)

2 tablespoons fresh lemon juice

2 tablespoons chopped mint

Remove the ends from the eggplants. Slice lengthwise into ¼–inch-thick slices. Trim the outside rounded sides of the eggplants so that they lie flat. Line a plate with paper towels and stack the eggplant slices on the plate, putting a paper towel between each layer. Cover the eggplant with another plate and weigh it down with a large, heavy can. Let the eggplant rest for 20 to 30 minutes to drain. Rinse and dry the eggplant.

Brush the vegetables with 2 tablespoons of the extra-virgin olive oil and sprinkle with ¼ teaspoon of the salt and ¼ teaspoon of the black pepper.

Heat an outdoor grill or an indoor grill pan to medium-high. If using an indoor grill pan, use 2 tablespoons of the extra-virgin olive oil to brush the pan as needed. If using an outdoor grill, use the 2 tablespoons extra-virgin olive oil to brush the vegetables as they cook. Grill the vegetables for 3 to 6 minutes on each side, until brown and softened. The peppers will take longer to cook. Transfer the grilled vegetables to a platter.

Combine the remaining 1 tablespoon of extra-virgin olive oil, the garlic, lemon juice, and remaining ¼ teaspoon salt and ¼ teaspoon black pepper. Pour over the vegetables and sprinkle with the mint.

Serve immediately, or for a more intense flavor allow the vegetables to marinate in the lemon dressing at room temperature for an hour or more.

Nutritional Analysis

Per serving: 143 Calories, 12 g Fat, 1.7 g Sat, 0 mg Chol,

4 g Fiber, 1.8 g Protein, 9 g Carb, 167 mg Sodium

Green Beans with Caramelized Red Onion

Bright green and crisp, these slender green beans are accented by sweet caramelized red onion. The beans and onion can both be prepared ahead and combined just before serving, making this a perfect side dish for a dinner party. If thin green beans are not available, substitute thicker, stringless green beans, sliced in half lengthwise.

Phase I: Detox
Gluten Free
Dairy Free
Vegetarian
Egg Free

1 pound whole thin green beans, stem ends trimmed

2 tablespoons extra-virgin olive oil

1 large (about 7- to 8-ounce) red onion, peeled, halved, and thinly sliced

½ teaspoon kosher salt

¼ teaspoon freshly ground black pepper

1 small clove garlic, minced

Serves 6
Serving size: ½ cup
Yield: 3 cups
Prep time: 10 minutes
Cook time: 35 minutes

Bring a large pan of salted water to a boil. Drop in the trimmed beans. Cook for about 1 to 2 minutes, until crisp-tender. Drain and immediately place in a bowl of ice water to cool. Drain and pat dry (this can be done ahead or while the onion is cooking).

Heat the extra-virgin olive oil in a large skillet over medium heat. Add the onion, salt, and pepper. Cook the onion for 10 to 15 minutes, or until translucent. Stir in the garlic, and continue to cook for about 20 minutes, until the onions are golden brown. Cover and reserve until ready to serve.

Just before serving, add the green beans to the onion. Warm thoroughly over medium heat and adjust seasonings.

Nutritional Analysis

Per ½-cup serving: 76 Calories, 5 g Fat, 0.7 g Sat, 0 mg Chol,

3 g Fiber, 2 g Protein, 8 g Carb, 165 mg Sodium

Herb-Roasted Butternut Squash with Shallots and Garlic

Phase I: Detox
Gluten Free
Dairy Free
Vegetarian
Egg Free

Serves 8
Serving size: ⅔ cup
Yield: 5 cups
Prep time: 20 minutes
Cook time: 40 to 45 minutes

The squash cooks soft in the center and slightly crispy on the outside, creating an earthy and satisfying dish. The roasted garlic is sweet, and pairs well with the squash and shallots.

1 medium (2½–3-pound) butternut squash, peeled and cut into 1-inch cubes

4 large shallots, peeled and cut in half

1 tablespoon minced rosemary

1 teaspoon minced thyme

¾ teaspoon kosher salt

½ teaspoon freshly ground black pepper

3 tablespoons plus 1 teaspoon extra-virgin olive oil

1 medium bulb garlic

Preheat the oven to 400 degrees F.

Place the squash, shallots, rosemary, thyme, salt, pepper, and 3 tablespoons of the extra-virgin olive oil on a large baking sheet. Stir to coat the squash and shallots with the olive oil and seasonings.

Cut the garlic across the top to remove the top ⅓ of the bulb. Drizzle the exposed garlic with the remaining 1 teaspoon of extra-virgin olive oil and sprinkle with salt and pepper. Wrap the garlic bulb in aluminum foil and place on the baking sheet with the squash.

Place the squash in the oven and roast for 20 minutes. Stir the squash and continue baking for another 20 to 25 minutes, or until the squash is soft and lightly browned.

Remove the garlic from the aluminum foil. Squeeze the individual cloves from the skin and stir them into the squash.

Nutritional Analysis

Per ⅔-cup serving: 124 Calories, 6 g Fat, 0.9 g Sat, 0 mg Chol,

3 g Fiber, 2 g Protein, 18 g Carb, 186 mg Sodium

Pan-Browned Brussels Sprouts

This is an easy and delicious treatment for these "little cabbages."

Phase I: Detox
Gluten Free
Dairy Free
Quick
Vegetarian
Egg Free

2 tablespoons extra-virgin olive oil

1 pound Brussels sprouts, trimmed and cut in half

½ teaspoon kosher salt

¼ teaspoon freshly ground black pepper

⅓ cup water

½ teaspoon lemon zest

Serves 4
Serving size: ¾ cup
Yield: 3 cups
Prep time: 10 minutes
Cook time: 10 minutes

Heat the extra-virgin olive oil in a medium skillet over medium-high heat. Add the Brussels sprouts, salt, and pepper and cook, stirring occasionally, for 2 or 3 minutes, until they begin to brown.

Add the water; cover the pan and cook for about 4 or 5 minutes, until almost done.

Remove the lid and turn the heat to high. Cook until brown and no liquid remains.

Sprinkle with the lemon zest.

Nutritional Analysis

Per ¾-cup serving: 107 Calories, 7 g Fat, 1.0 g Sat, 0 mg Chol, 4 g Fiber, 3 g Protein, 9 g Carb, 266 mg Sodium

Ratatouille

Phase I: Detox
Gluten Free
Dairy Free
Vegetarian
Egg Free

Serves 8
Serving size: ½ cup
Yield: 4 cups
Prep time: 30 minutes
Cook time: 1½ hours
(unattended time about
1 hour)

This is the classic mix of eggplant, zucchini, red peppers, and tomatoes, but the fresh herbs stirred in at the end of the cooking process set this version apart. Good served hot or at room temperature, drizzled with a touch of olive oil, ratatouille travels well and tastes even better the day after it's made.

1 medium eggplant (about 12 ounces), cut into ¾-inch cubes

¾ teaspoon kosher salt

4 tablespoons extra-virgin olive oil

2 medium yellow onions, peeled and cut into ½-inch pieces

2 medium cloves garlic, minced (about 2 teaspoons)

2 medium red bell peppers (6 ounces each), cored, seeded, and cut into ¾-inch pieces

2 small zucchini (about 12 ounces), cut into ¾-inch pieces

1½ cups coarsely chopped tomato

1 large sprig of thyme

½ teaspoon freshly ground black pepper

¼ cup shredded basil

¼ cup finely chopped parsley

Sprinkle the eggplant cubes with ¼ teaspoon of the salt and place the eggplant in a colander set over a bowl. Cover the eggplant with a paper towel and place a

The UltraMetabolism Cookbook

plate over the towel. Weigh the plate down with a heavy can to press down on the eggplant. Let the eggplant drain for about 30 minutes to extract any bitter juice. After the eggplant has drained, rinse it and pat dry with paper towels.

Heat 2 tablespoons of the extra-virgin olive oil in a medium skillet over medium heat. Add the onion and ¼ teaspoon of the salt. Cook the onion for about 3 minutes, until translucent and beginning to soften. Add the garlic and cook for 1 to 2 minutes, until the garlic and onion are lightly browned. Remove the garlic and onion with a slotted spoon and place them in a medium Dutch oven or casserole.

Add 1 more tablespoon of the extra-virgin olive oil to the skillet. Stir in the peppers and ¼ teaspoon of the salt and cook for about 7 minutes, until the peppers are just beginning to brown.

Using a slotted spoon, transfer the peppers from the skillet to the Dutch oven or casserole. Add the zucchini and cook for about 4 minutes. Remove the zucchini from the skillet with the slotted spoon and add it to the Dutch oven or casserole.

Add the remaining 1 tablespoon of extra-virgin olive oil to the skillet and cook the eggplant, stirring occasionally. When lightly browned, add it to the Dutch oven or casserole.

Add the tomatoes to the skillet. Scrape up any browned bits on the bottom of the skillet. Add the tomatoes to the Dutch oven or casserole, along with the thyme and black pepper. Bring the vegetables to a simmer. Cover and cook, stirring occasionally, for about 45 minutes.

Remove the lid and continue cooking for about 15 minutes. When done, the vegetables should be soft and the sauce thick. Stir in the basil and parsley. Serve hot or at room temperature.

Nutritional Analysis

Per ½-cup serving: 119 Calories, 9.3 g Fat, 1.4 g Sat, 2 mg Chol, 4 g Fiber, 3 g Protein, 12 g Carb, 267 mg Sodium

Roasted Peppers

Any peppers, from the tiniest serranos, to poblanos, and of course large bell peppers, can be roasted. Roasting gives peppers a sweeter taste and a somewhat smoky flavor. Any juice that accumulates while peeling the peppers is tasty, and can be poured over the peppers.

Phase I: Detox
Gluten Free
Dairy Free
Quick
Vegetarian
Egg Free

Serves 4
Serving size: ½ cup
Yield: 2 cups
Prep time: 10 minutes
Cook time: 10 minutes

4 medium red bell peppers (about 5 to 6 ounces each)

Broiler method: Preheat the broiler to high. Lay the peppers on a sheet pan and place under the broiler 2 to 3 inches from the element. Cook, turning with tongs, until charred on all sides.

Stovetop method: Place the whole peppers directly on the gas flame, turning with tongs until charred on all sides.

Outdoor grill method: Preheat the grill to high. Lay the whole peppers in the grill grate and cook, turning with tongs, until charred on all sides.

Place the charred peppers in a bowl and cover tightly with plastic wrap, or place in a large saucepan with a tight-fitting lid. When the peppers are cool enough to handle, remove the charred skin, the core, and the seeds. The skin should come off easily. Do not run the peppers under water, as this will decrease their flavor. Peel over a plate and save any juices that drain from the peppers. Pour the juice over the peeled peppers.

Store refrigerated in a closed container for up to 5 days, or freeze in a zip-top freezer bag.

Nutritional Analysis

Per ½-cup serving: 31 Calories, 0 g Fat, 0 g Sat, 0 mg Chol, 2 g Fiber, 1 g Protein, 7 g Carb, 2 mg Sodium

Roasted Red Potatoes with Rosemary

Quick and easy, these flavorful potatoes complement any meat, fish, or poultry.

1 pound (about 16) small red potatoes, cut into quarters

3 tablespoons extra-virgin olive oil

1 tablespoon chopped rosemary

½ teaspoon kosher salt

½ teaspoon freshly ground black pepper

Preheat the oven to 400 degrees F.

Toss together the potatoes, extra-virgin olive oil, rosemary, salt, and pepper. Spread the potatoes on a baking sheet. Roast for about 20 to 25 minutes, until the potatoes are golden on the outside and soft in the center.

Phase I: Detox
Gluten Free
Dairy Free
Quick
Vegetarian
Egg Free

Serves 4
Serving size: ⅔ cup
Yield: 2⅔ cups
Prep time: 5 minutes
Cook time: 20 to 25 minutes

Nutritional Analysis

Per ⅔-cup serving: 176 Calories, 11 g Fat, 1.5 g Sat, 0 mg Chol,

1.9 g Fiber, 2 g Protein, 18 g Carb, 247 mg Sodium

Sautéed Broccoli Rabe with Garlic and Pine Nuts

This is a classic combination of sautéed sliced garlic and bitter greens. Because of the blanching and quick sauté, the broccoli rabe retains its vibrant green color. The red pepper flakes add a slight bit of heat, and the toasted pine nuts add crunch. This side dish pairs well with grilled meats and poultry.

2 pounds broccoli rabe, tough stems removed, coarsely chopped (about 12 cups)

2 tablespoons pine nuts

¼ cup extra-virgin olive oil

6 medium cloves garlic, thinly sliced

¼ teaspoon crushed red pepper flakes

¼ teaspoon kosher salt

Phase I: Detox
Gluten Free
Dairy Free
Quick
Vegetarian
Egg Free

Serves 4
Serving size: 1 cup
Yield: 4 cups
Prep time: 15 minutes
Cook time: 10 minutes

Bring a large pot of salted water to a boil. Drop in the chopped broccoli rabe and cook for 1 minute, until it wilts. Immediately drain, and place in a bowl of ice water to cool. Drain and set aside.

Meanwhile, toast the pine nuts in a small skillet over medium heat for about 3 to 4 minutes, until lightly browned. Stir the pine nuts frequently and watch closely to prevent burning. When toasted, remove the nuts to a plate to cool.

Heat the extra-virgin olive oil in a large skillet over medium-high heat. Add the garlic and cook, stirring, until golden. Add the broccoli rabe, red pepper flakes, and salt and cook until tender and heated through.

Adjust the seasoning if necessary. Add the pine nuts and serve.

Nutritional Analysis

Per 1-cup serving: 228 Calories, 17 g Fat, 2 g Sat, 0 mg Chol,

0.3 g Fiber, 9 g Protein, 13 g Carb, 188 mg Sodium

Sautéed Spinach with Garlic and Lemon

Phase I: Detox
Gluten Free
Dairy Free
Quick
Vegetarian
Egg Free

Serves 4
Serving size: ½ cup
Yield: 2 cups
Prep time: 15 minutes
Cook time: 5 to 8 minutes

Serve meat, fish, or poultry atop a bed of this simple, delicious, bright green spinach.

3 tablespoons extra-virgin olive oil

4 medium cloves garlic, chopped

2 bunches fresh spinach (about 2 pounds), thoroughly washed

½ teaspoon kosher salt

½ teaspoon freshly ground black pepper

Zest of 1 lemon (about ½ teaspoon)

Heat the extra-virgin olive oil in a large skillet over medium heat. Add the garlic and cook until golden. Add the spinach, salt, and pepper. Cook, turning the spinach in the pan, until the spinach is wilted. Remove from the heat and stir in the lemon zest.

Nutritional Analysis

Per ½-cup serving: 136 Calories, 11 g Fat, 1.6 g Sat, 0 mg Chol, 4 g Fiber, 5 g Protein, 7 g Carb, 370 mg Sodium

Simple Steamed Artichokes

Artichokes are fun for the entire family to eat. This simple method of cooking makes the artichokes compatible with many of the sauces in this book. They are especially tasty with Herbed Lemon Dipping Sauce (page 169).

4 large artichokes, leaves and stem trimmed, cut surfaces rubbed with fresh lemon
½ teaspoon kosher salt

Phase I: Detox
Gluten Free
Dairy Free
Vegetarian
Egg Free

Serves 4
Serving size: 1 artichoke
Yield: 4 artichokes
Prep time: 10 minutes
Cook time: 25 to 30 minutes

Place the artichokes upside down on a steaming rack over boiling water. Cook for 25 to 30 minutes, or until a leaf pulls out easily from the artichoke and the bottom is tender when pierced with a small knife or fork. Place the cooked artichoke in a bowl of ice water or rinse under cold water to stop the cooking. Transfer to a plate and place upside down to drain.

Alternatively, place the artichokes in a pot or deep sauté pan large enough to hold them in a single layer. Put 1 inch of boiling water in the pot with ½ teaspoon salt. Bring to a simmer and cook the artichokes, covered, for 25 to 30 minutes. Proceed as above with the steaming method.

Serve cold or at room temperature with Herbed Lemon Dipping Sauce (page 169), if desired.

Nutritional Analysis

Per artichoke: 85 Calories, 0 g Fat, 0 g Sat, 0 mg Chol, 10 g Fiber, 7 g Protein, 20 g Carb, 255 mg Sodium

Slivered Brussels Sprouts with Shiitake Mushrooms

A perfect side dish for fall, with the fall colors of green, gold, and brown.

Phase I: Detox
Gluten Free
Dairy Free
Vegetarian
Egg Free

Serves 6
Serving size: ½ cup
Yield: 3 cups
Prep time: 30 minutes
Cook time: 20 minutes

1 pound Brussels sprouts

½ pound shiitake mushrooms

5 tablespoons extra-virgin olive oil

3 tablespoons minced shallot (about 1 ounce)

1 teaspoon minced garlic (about 1 medium clove)

½ teaspoon kosher salt

1 large sprig of thyme

½ teaspoon lemon zest

2 teaspoons fresh lemon juice

Trim the Brussels sprouts and cut them in half lengthwise. Cut each half horizontally into thin slivers.

Clean the mushrooms with a damp paper towel. Remove the stems and slice the caps into ¼-inch-thick slices.

Heat 3 tablespoons of the extra-virgin olive oil in a large skillet over medium-high heat. Add the shallot and cook, stirring, for about 2 minutes, until translucent. Add the garlic, ½ teaspoon of the salt, the thyme, and sliced mushrooms. Cook the mushrooms for about 7 minutes, until they have given up their liquid and are lightly browned. Remove the mushrooms from the skillet to a plate.

In the same skillet, heat the remaining 2 tablespoons of extra-virgin olive oil. Add the Brussels sprouts, flat side down, and the remaining ½ teaspoon salt. Cook over medium-high heat for about 8 minutes, until the Brussels sprouts have softened and are beginning to brown. Stir in the mushrooms and heat thoroughly over medium heat. Add the lemon juice and lemon zest before serving.

Nutritional Analysis

Per ½-cup serving: 160 Calories, 12 g Fat, 1.7 g Sat, 0 mg Chol, 3 g Fiber, 3 g Protein, 13 g Carb, 179 mg Sodium

Slow-Roasted Russet Potatoes with Oregano and Garlic

These are golden brown and crispy on the outside and soft on the inside. The taste of the oregano is subtle but adds another dimension of flavor. This is perfect dish to prepare for guests, because the potatoes roast unattended, freeing up time to prepare another part of the meal.

Phase I: Detox
Gluten Free
Dairy Free
Vegetarian
Egg Free

Serves 4
Serving size: 1 potato
Yield: 4 potatoes
Prep time: 15 minutes
Cook time: 1½ hours

4 medium russet potatoes (about 1½ pounds), cut into quarters

3 tablespoons extra-virgin olive oil

1 teaspoon minced garlic (about 1 medium clove)

1 tablespoon minced oregano

1 teaspoon kosher salt

½ teaspoon freshly ground black pepper

Preheat the oven to 350 degrees F.

Bring 4 cups of water to a boil in a medium pot. Add the potatoes. Return the water to a boil and cook the potatoes for 2 minutes. Remove the potatoes from the water and place in a shallow roasting pan in a single layer.

Add the extra-virgin olive oil, garlic, oregano, salt, and pepper.

Roast for about 1½ hours, until golden brown. Turn the potatoes every 30 minutes while baking.

Nutritional Analysis

Per potato: 155 Calories, 4 g Fat, 0.5 g Sat, 0 mg Chol, 3 g Fiber, 3 g Protein, 29 g Carb, 487 mg Sodium

Stir-Fried Edamame

Phase I: Detox
Gluten Free
Dairy Free
Quick
Vegetarian
Egg Free

Serves 4
Serving size: ¾ cup
Yield: 3 cups
Prep time: 10 minutes
Cook time: 6 minutes

This crisp, stir-fried edamame is a very spicy dish, but the red chili paste can be reduced for those who prefer less heat. No need to defrost the edamame—use them right from the freezer for a quick and easy side dish for virtually any meal.

2 teaspoons dark sesame oil

1 teaspoon light sesame oil

1 teaspoon minced garlic

1 teaspoon minced ginger

1 (10-ounce) package frozen shelled edamame

1 tablespoon low-sodium wheat-free tamari

1 teaspoon rice wine vinegar

¼ teaspoon Thai Kitchen Red Chili Paste

2 medium scallions, thinly sliced

2 teaspoons sesame seeds

Heat the dark and light sesame oil in a medium skillet over medium–high heat. Add the garlic and ginger, and cook for 1 minute. Stir in the edamame and stir quickly for 1 to 2 minutes, until the edamame begin to turn bright green and soften. Add the tamari, rice wine vinegar, and red chili paste and cook for 2 minutes. Stir in the scallions and sesame seeds just before serving.

Nutritional Analysis

Per ¾-cup serving: 139 Calories, 7 g Fat, 0.5 g Sat, 0 mg Chol, 4 g Fiber, 8 g Protein, 10 g Carb, 400 mg Sodium

Sweet Potato-Carrot Mash

This smooth vegetable purée has a creamy texture, despite the fact that it contains no cream.

4 medium sweet potatoes (about 1¾ pounds)

1 pound carrots, peeled and cut into 1-inch chunks

2 tablespoons plus 1 teaspoon extra-virgin olive oil

½ teaspoon kosher salt

Pinch of ground red pepper

Pinch of freshly ground or grated nutmeg

Pinch of freshly ground black pepper

Phase I: Detox
Gluten Free
Dairy Free
Vegetarian
Egg Free

Serves 4
Serving size: ⅔ cup
Yield: 2⅔ cups
Prep time: 15 minutes
Cook time: 50 minutes

Preheat the oven to 425 degrees F.

Pierce the sweet potatoes with a knife in about 3 places.

Place the carrots on a baking sheet. Mix with 1 tablespoon of the extra-virgin olive oil and ¼ teaspoon of the salt.

Place the sweet potatoes and carrots in the oven. Bake until the potatoes and carrots are soft when pierced with a fork, about 40 minutes for the carrots and 50 minutes for the sweet potatoes. Turn carrots once while cooking.

When cool enough to handle, peel the sweet potatoes and place them in the bowl of a food processor with the carrots. Add the extra-virgin olive oil, ground red pepper, nutmeg, black pepper, and the remaining ¼ teaspoon salt. Process until smooth.

Nutritional Analysis

Per ⅔-cup serving: 232 Calories, 8 g Fat, 1.2 g Sat, 0 mg Chol,

7 g Fiber, 4 g Protein, 37 g Carb, 335 mg Sodium

Wild Mushroom Sauté

Phase I: Detox
Gluten Free
Dairy Free
Quick
Vegetarian
Egg Free

Serves 8
Serving size: scant ½ cup
Yield: 3½ cups
Prep time: 20 minutes
Cook time: 15 minutes

The mushrooms' rich brown color and flavor are deeply satisfying. Shiitake, cremini, or oyster mushrooms, alone or in combination, work best for this dish.

4 tablespoons extra-virgin olive oil

3 medium shallots, peeled and minced (about 3 tablespoons)

2 large cloves garlic, minced (about 1 tablespoon)

2 pounds wild mushrooms, cleaned, stems removed, sliced ¼-inch thick

3 multibranch sprigs of thyme

1 bay leaf

½ teaspoon kosher salt

½ teaspoon freshly ground black pepper

2 tablespoons minced parsley

Heat the extra-virgin olive oil in a large skillet over medium-high heat. Add the shallots and cook, stirring for about 3 to 4 minutes, until translucent. Add the garlic and cook for about 1 minute, until fragrant.

Add the mushrooms, thyme, and bay leaf and cook, stirring occasionally, until the mushrooms have released their juice. Season with the salt and pepper and cook for about 5 minutes more, until the mushrooms have browned. Remove and discard the bay leaf.

Sprinkle with the minced parsley and serve.

Nutritional Analysis

Per scant ½-cup serving: 108 Calories, 7.5 g Fat, 1.0 g Sat, 0 mg Chol,

2 g Fiber, 4 g Protein, 9 g Carb, 139 mg Sodium

Lime-Scented Coconut Rice

Coconut milk adds richness, fresh lime juice adds tang, and the toasted cashews provide crunch. The confetti-like appearance comes from the flecks of green scallion and cilantro.

2 tablespoons extra-virgin olive oil

2 tablespoons minced onion

1 teaspoon minced garlic

1 cup brown basmati rice

¾ cup organic low-sodium chicken or vegetable broth

¾ cup canned unsweetened lite coconut milk

½ cup water

½ teaspoon kosher salt

¼ cup finely chopped raw, unsalted cashews

½ cup thinly sliced scallions

¼ cup minced cilantro

1 tablespoon fresh lime juice

Phase I: Detox
Gluten Free
Dairy Free
Vegetarian (with vegetable broth)
Egg Free

Serves 6
Serving size: ½ cup
Yield: 3 cups
Prep time: 20 minutes
Cook time: 45 minutes

Heat the extra-virgin olive oil in a medium saucepan over medium-high heat. Add the onion and cook, stirring, for about 3 minutes, until translucent. Add the garlic and cook, stirring, for 30 seconds. Stir in the rice and coat it with the oil. Add the broth, coconut milk, water, and salt. Bring to a simmer, cover, and cook for 40 to 60 minutes, until the liquid is absorbed. The cooking time of the rice may vary. Turn off the heat and let the rice sit for 5 minutes.

Meanwhile, toast the cashews in a small skillet over medium-low heat for about 5 minutes, until lightly colored. Stir frequently and watch closely to prevent burning. When toasted, remove the cashews to a plate to cool.

When the rice is done, fluff it with a fork. Stir in the scallions, cilantro, and lime juice. Serve garnished with the toasted cashews.

Nutritional Analysis

Per ½-cup serving: 216 Calories, 9.5 g Fat, 5.0 g Sat, 1 mg Chol, 2 g Fiber, 5 g Pro, 28 g Carb, 186 mg Sodium

Roasted Sweet Potatoes

Phase I: Detox
Gluten Free
Dairy Free
Vegetarian
Egg Free

Serves 4
Serving size: generous
¾ cup
Yield: 3½ cups
Prep time: 10 minutes
Cook time: 40 minutes

A perfect side dish for the fall or winter—the soft and slightly browned sweet potatoes are enhanced by the spices, while the salt and pepper provide contrast to the sweetness of the potatoes.

4 large (about 2¼ pounds) sweet potatoes, peeled and each cut into 8 pieces

3 tablespoons extra-virgin olive oil

½ teaspoon kosher salt

½ teaspoon freshly ground black pepper

¼ teaspoon ground red pepper

¼ teaspoon ground cinnamon

2 tablespoons snipped chives

Kosher salt to taste (optional)

Preheat the oven to 425 degrees F.

Place the potatoes on a large baking sheet. Drizzle with the extra-virgin olive oil, salt, black pepper, red pepper, and cinnamon. Toss to combine the ingredients.

Bake for about 40 minutes, until brown and soft, turning twice during cooking.

Sprinkle with the chives and kosher salt, if desired.

Nutritional Analysis

Per ¾-cup serving: 217 Calories, 11 g Fat, 1.5 g Sat, 0 mg Chol,

5 g Fiber, 3 g Protein, 36 g Carb, 294 mg Sodium

Hot Buckwheat, Banana, Flax, and Walnuts

Phase I: Detox
Gluten Free
Dairy Free
Quick
Vegetarian
Egg Free

Serves 4
Serving size: ⅔ cup
Yield: 2⅔ cups
Prep time: 5 minutes
Cook time: 25 minutes

This is a creamy, hot breakfast cereal.

1 cup buckwheat groats, whole (kasha)
2 cups plain soy milk
¼ teaspoon ground cinnamon
Pinch kosher salt (optional)
1 small banana, mashed
2 tablespoons flaxseed, ground
2 tablespoons chopped walnuts

Place the buckwheat, soy milk, cinnamon, salt, and mashed banana in a medium saucepan. Bring to a boil, stirring frequently. Cover the pan and reduce heat to low. Simmer for 15 to 20 minutes, until the buckwheat is tender. Top with ground flaxseeds and chopped walnuts.

Nutritional Analysis

Per ⅔ -cup serving: 270 Calories, 8 g Fat, .08 g Sat, 0 g Chol, 7 g Fiber, 12 g Protein, 43 g Carb, 55 mg Sodium

Crispy Pan-Roasted Red Potatoes

Because these already tiny potatoes are cut small, they crisp all over. Very versatile, they can accompany any meat, poultry, or fish.

¼ cup extra-virgin olive oil

1½ pounds red potatoes, cut into ½-inch dice

½ teaspoon kosher salt

½ teaspoon freshly ground black pepper

1 tablespoon snipped chives

Heat the extra-virgin olive oil in a large skillet over medium-high heat. Add the potatoes and turn to coat them in the oil. Sprinkle the potatoes with the salt. Cook, stirring occasionally, for about 25 minutes. The potatoes are done when they are crisp and brown on the outside and soft inside. If the potatoes are browning too quickly, reduce the heat.

When done, sprinkle the potatoes with the black pepper and chives before serving.

Phase I: Detox
Gluten Free
Dairy Free
Vegetarian
Egg Free

Serves 4
Serving size: ⅔ cup
Yield: 2⅔ cups
Prep time: 10 minutes
Cook time: 25 minutes

Nutritional Analysis

Per ⅔-cup serving: 249 Calories, 14 g Fat, 2.0 g Sat, 0 mg Chol,

3 g Fiber, 3 g Protein, 27 g Carb, 240 mg Sodium

Apple-Walnut Amaranth

Amaranth is a nutty, nutritious grain full of vitamins, minerals, and protein.

1 cup amaranth

3 cups plain soy milk

¼ teaspoon ground cinnamon

Pinch kosher salt (optional)

1 large apple, skin on, cored and diced

½ cup chopped walnuts

Phase I: Detox
Gluten Free
Dairy Free
Vegetarian
Egg Free

Serves 4
Serving size: ⅔ cup
Yield: 2⅔ cups
Prep time: 5 minutes
Cook time: 30 minutes

Place the amaranth, soy milk, cinnamon, salt (if using), and apple in a medium saucepan. Bring to a boil, stirring frequently. Cover pan and reduce heat to low. Simmer for 25 to 30 minutes until amaranth is soft. Top with chopped walnuts and serve.

Nutritional Analysis

Per ⅔-cup serving: 380 Calories, 15 g Fat, 2.2 g Sat, 0 mg Chol, 10 g Fiber, 16 g Protein, 48 g Carb, 83 mg Sodium

Berriest Smoothie

A quick, easy breakfast smoothie.

½ cup plain soy milk

½ cup plain soy yogurt

1½ cups fresh or frozen mixed berries

1 tablespoon flaxseed, ground

Phase I: Detox
Gluten Free
Dairy Free
Quick
Vegetarian
Egg Free

Serves 1
Serving size: 2½ cups
Yield: 2½ cups
Prep time: 5 minutes
Cook time: none

Place all the ingredients in a blender and mix until smooth.

Nutritional Analysis

Per 2½-cup serving: 287 Calories, 8 g Fat, 1.1 g Sat, 0 mg Chol, 10 g Fiber, 10 g Protein, 48 g Carb, 80 mg Sodium

Peach Quinoa with Flax and Nuts

Phase I: Detox
Gluten Free
Dairy Free
Quick
Vegetarian
Egg Free

Serves 4
Serving size: ¾ cup
Yield: 3 cups
Prep time: 5 minutes
Cook time: 25 minutes

The South American grain, quinoa, along with flaxseed serves up plenty of protein and healthful omega-3 fats.

1 cup quinoa, thoroughly rinsed and drained

2 cups plain soy milk

¼ teaspoon ground allspice

Pinch kosher salt (optional)

2 medium peaches, peeled, pitted, and diced, or 1½ cups frozen peaches

2 tablespoons flaxseed, ground

2 tablespoons chopped hazelnuts

Place the quinoa, soy milk, allspice, salt (if using), and peaches in a medium saucepan. Bring to a boil, stirring frequently. Cover pan and simmer on low heat for approximately 20 minutes, until quinoa is tender. Top with ground flaxseed and chopped hazelnuts.

Nutritional Analysis

Per ¾-cup serving: 285 Calories, 9 g Fat, 1 g Sat, 0 mg Chol, 5 g Fiber, 12 g Protein, 41 g Carb, 59 mg Sodium

Hot Brown Rice, Nuts, and Flax

Phase I: Detox
Gluten Free
Dairy Free
Quick
Vegetarian
Egg Free

Serves 2
Serving size: ¾ cup
Yield: 1½ cups
Prep time: 5 minutes
Cook time: 50 minutes

A way to eat brown rice for breakfast.

½ cup long-grain brown rice

1 cup plain soy milk

¼ teaspoon ground nutmeg

Pinch kosher salt (optional)

8 Brazil nuts, shelled and chopped

2 tablespoons flaxseed, ground

Place the brown rice, soy milk, nutmeg, and salt (if using) in a medium saucepan. Bring to a boil, stirring frequently. Cover pan and reduce the heat to low. Simmer for approximately 45 minutes. Top with chopped Brazil nuts and ground flaxseed.

Nutritional Analysis

Per ¾-cup serving: 372 Calories, 17 g Fat, 3.2 g Sat, 0 mg Chol, 6 g Fiber, 12 g Protein, 46 g Carb, 56 mg Sodium

Turkey Breakfast Sausage

This flavorful breakfast sausage with sage and apple is a delicious, healthy alternative to store-bought sausage.

Phase I: Detox
Gluten Free
Dairy Free
Quick
Egg Free

Serves 8
Serving size: 1 (2-ounce)
patty
Yield: 8 patties
Prep time: 20 minutes
Cook time: 6 to 8 minutes

1 pound ground turkey breast

¼ cup finely diced apple, such as Gala or Red Delicious

2 tablespoons finely minced red onion

2 teaspoons finely minced sage

½ teaspoon finely minced thyme

3 tablespoons extra-virgin olive oil

½ teaspoon kosher salt

½ teaspoon freshly ground black pepper

In a large bowl, gently mix together the ground turkey, apple, onion, sage, thyme, 1 tablespoon of the extra-virgin olive oil, the salt, and pepper. Form the mixture into eight 4-inch patties, each about ½ inch thick.

Heat the remaining 2 tablespoons of extra-virgin olive oil in a nonstick skillet over medium heat. Cook the patties for 3 to 4 minutes on each side, until firm to the touch.

Nutritional Analysis

Per 2-ounce patty: 126 Calories, 9 g Fat, 1.7 g Sat, 33 mg Chol,

0 g Fiber, 11 g Protein, 1 g Carb, 160 mg Sodium

Yogurt with Fresh Fruit, Shredded Coconut, and Wheat Germ

Phase I: Detox
Gluten Free
Dairy Free
Quick
Vegetarian
Egg Free

Serves 1
Serving size: 2 cups
Yield: 2 cups
Prep time: 5 minutes
Cook time: none

8 ounces plain nonfat soy yogurt

1 cup fruit in season: kiwi, strawberries, mango, diced

2 teaspoons grated coconut

1 teaspoon raw wheat germ

Mix fruit in yogurt and top with grated coconut and wheat germ.

Nutritional Analysis

Per 2-cup serving: 275 Calories, 5 g Fat, 1.9 g Sat, 5 mg Chol,

5 g Fiber, 17 g Protein, 43 g Carb, 194 mg Sodium

Basic Tomato Salsa

Use the ripest, juiciest tomatoes available for a fresh, flavorful salsa. Serve with sliced vegetables or as a sauce for grilled fish or chicken.

1 cup chopped tomatoes (about 6 ounces)

3 tablespoons finely minced cilantro

2 tablespoons finely minced red onion

2 teaspoons fresh lime juice

1 teaspoon minced jalapeño pepper

¼ teaspoon kosher salt

¼ teaspoon freshly ground black pepper

Phase I: Detox
Gluten Free
Dairy Free
Quick
Vegetarian
Egg Free

Serves 4
Serving size: ¼ cup
Yield: 1 cup
Prep time: 15 minutes
Cook time: none

In a medium bowl, mix all ingredients together. Serve chilled or at room temperature.

Nutritional Analysis

Per ¼-cup serving: 13 Calories, 0 g Fat, 0 g Sat, 0 mg Chol, 0.4 g Fiber, 0 g Protein, 3 g Carb, 122 mg Sodium

Basil Pesto

This is a classic dairy-free pesto with a vibrant green color, perfect as a fresh finishing touch for sauces, salad dressings, or dips.

3 cups loosely packed fresh basil leaves

½ cup extra-virgin olive oil

1 large clove garlic, chopped

2 tablespoons pine nuts

½ teaspoon kosher salt

Phase I: Detox
Gluten Free
Dairy Free
Quick
Vegetarian
Egg Free

Serves 12
Serving size: 1 tablespoon
Yield: ¾ cup
Prep time: 10 minutes
Cook time: none

Combine all ingredients in the bowl of a food processor and pulse until smooth.

To freeze pesto: Pour the pesto into ice cube trays. Freeze. Remove the pesto cubes from the tray and store them in a zip-top bag. Thaw and use the pesto as needed.

Nutritional Analysis

Per 1-tablespoon serving: 93 Calories, 10 g Fat, 1.4 g Sat, 0 mg Chol,

0 g Fiber, 0 g Protein, 1 g Carb, 80 mg Sodium

Cilantro Pesto

Phase I: Detox
Gluten Free
Dairy Free
Quick
Vegetarian
Egg Free

Serves 5
Serving size: 2 tablespoons
Yield: about ⅔ cup
Prep time: 10 minutes
Cook time: none

A delicious twist on the traditional basil sauce, this pesto is great on grilled fish or chicken.

4 cups cilantro leaves and tender stems, roughly chopped

2 medium cloves garlic, roughly chopped

¼ cup extra-virgin olive oil

4 teaspoons fresh lime juice

½ teaspoon kosher salt

¼ teaspoon freshly ground black pepper

½ teaspoon minced jalapeño pepper

Combine all ingredients in the bowl of a food processor fitted with a metal blade and process until smooth.

Nutritional Analysis

Per 2-tablespoon serving: 107 Calories, 11 g Fat, 1.6 g Sat, 0 mg Chol,

0 g Fiber, 0 g Protein, 1 g Carb, 198 mg Sodium

Herbed Lemon Dipping Sauce

Full of fresh lemon and herb flavor, this makes a wonderful dipping sauce for artichokes. It's also good drizzled over plain grilled fish, white-meat poultry, or seafood.

½ teaspoon lemon zest

2 tablespoons fresh lemon juice

1½ teaspoons minced garlic (about 1 large clove)

2 teaspoons minced parsley

2 teaspoons minced tarragon

2 teaspoons minced chives

2 teaspoons minced mint leaves

½ teaspoon kosher salt

¼ teaspoon freshly ground black pepper

6 tablespoons extra-virgin olive oil

Phase I: Detox
Gluten Free
Dairy Free
Quick
Vegetarian
Egg Free

Serves 4
Serving size: 2 tablespoons
Yield: ½ cup
Prep time: 10 minutes
Cook time: none

In a small bowl, whisk together the lemon zest, lemon juice, garlic, parsley, tarragon, chives, mint, salt, and pepper. Slowly whisk in the extra-virgin olive oil until slightly thickened. Alternatively, place the ingredients in a jar with a tight-fitting lid and shake well to combine.

Nutritional Analysis

Per 2-tablespoon serving: 194 Calories, 21 g Fat, 2.9 g Sat, 0 mg Chol,

0 g Fiber, 0 g Protein, 1 g Carb, 242 mg Sodium

Herbed Tomato Sauce

Phase I: Detox
Gluten Free
Dairy Free
Quick
Vegetarian
Egg Free

Serves: 7
Serving size: ⅓ cup
Yield: 2⅓ cups
Prep time: 10 minutes
Cook time: 20 to 25 minutes

This is a somewhat spicy sauce, with the fresh taste and antioxidant power of oregano, parsley, and basil.

¼ cup extra-virgin olive oil

1 medium clove garlic, minced

1 (28-ounce) can low-sodium whole tomatoes, drained

1 tablespoon finely chopped flat-leaf parsley

1 teaspoon finely chopped oregano

½ teaspoon kosher salt

¼ teaspoon crushed red pepper flakes

¼ teaspoon freshly ground black pepper

6 fresh basil leaves, cut in thin strips (about 2 tablespoons)

Heat the extra-virgin olive oil in a medium saucepan. Add the garlic and cook for 1 to 2 minutes, until golden. Add the tomatoes, crushing them by hand as they are stirred into the garlic and olive oil. Stir in the parsley, oregano, salt, red pepper flakes, and black pepper. Bring to a simmer and cook for about 20 minutes, until the sauce has thickened. Stir in the basil.

Nutritional Analysis

Per ⅓-cup serving: 108 Calories, 9 g Fat, 1.3 g Sat, 0 mg Chol, 1 g Fiber, 2 g Protein, 5 g Carb, 283 mg Sodium

Mango Salsa

Serve this sweet, tart, spicy, and refreshing salsa with grilled fish, Grilled Shrimp Brochettes (page 97), or chicken.

1 mango, peeled, pitted, and diced

4 teaspoons fresh lime juice

1 tablespoon minced red onion

1 tablespoon minced cilantro

1 teaspoon minced jalapeño pepper

Pinch of kosher salt

Pinch of freshly ground black pepper

In a small bowl, gently stir together all ingredients.

Nutritional Analysis

Per ¼-cup serving: 48 Calories, 0 g Fat, 0 g Sat, 0 mg Chol, 1.3 g Fiber, 0.5 g Protein, 13 g Carb, 82 mg Sodium

Phase I: Detox
Gluten Free
Dairy Free
Quick
Vegetarian
Egg Free

Serves 3
Serving size: ¼ cup
Yield: ¾ cup
Prep time: 15 minutes
Cook time: none

Mediterranean Tomato Salsa

Phase I: Detox
Gluten Free
Dairy Free
Quick
Vegetarian
Egg Free

Serves 6
Serving size: ¼ cup
Yield: 1½ cups
Prep time: 25 minutes
Cook time: none

Briny olives, capers, fresh herbs, pine nuts, and of course, the most flavorful tomatoes available make this salsa explode with Mediterranean flavors. In the winter use grape tomatoes for the best flavor, and in the summer, fresh local tomatoes are choice. Kalamatas are suggested for the olives.

1 cup chopped tomato

5 tablespoons chopped brine-cured black olives

3 tablespoons minced basil (about 4 to 5 large leaves)

2 tablespoons minced parsley

1 tablespoon minced red onion

1 teaspoon minced garlic

2 tablespoons extra-virgin olive oil

1 tablespoon drained capers

1 tablespoon pine nuts

½ teaspoon fresh lemon juice

¼ teaspoon kosher salt

¼ teaspoon freshly ground black pepper

In a medium bowl, stir all ingredients together well to combine.

Nutritional Analysis

Per ¼-cup serving: 68 Calories, 6 g Fat, 0.8 g Sat, 0 mg Chol, 1 g Fiber, 1 g Protein, 2 g Carb, 186 mg Sodium

Tahini Dressing

Serve on Asian Chicken Salad (page 96), as a dip with fresh raw vegetables, or on shredded pork.

½ cup tahini

½ cup light sesame oil

2 teaspoons minced garlic (about 2 medium cloves)

½ teaspoon grated fresh ginger

3 tablespoons fresh lemon juice

3 tablespoons low-sodium wheat-free tamari

1 tablespoon dark sesame oil

½ teaspoon kosher salt

½ teaspoon Thai Kitchen Red Chili Paste

Combine the tahini, light sesame oil, garlic, ginger, lemon juice, tamari, dark sesame oil, salt, and red chili paste in the bowl of a food processor fitted with a metal blade. Process just until smooth. If the dressing seems too thick, add a little water.

Nutritional Analysis

Per 2-tablespoon serving: 157 Calories, 17 g Fat, 2.3 g Sat, 0 mg Chol,

0 g Fiber, 3 g Protein, 1.5 g Carb, 240 mg Sodium

Phase I: Detox
Gluten Free
Dairy Free
Quick
Vegetarian
Egg Free

Serves 12
Serving size: 2 tablespoons
Yield 1½ cups
Prep time: 10 minutes
Cook time: none

Vinaigrettes, Sauces, and Dressings

Basic Vinaigrette

Phase I: Detox
Gluten Free
Dairy Free
Quick
Vegetarian
Egg Free

Serves 4
Serving size: 2 tablespoons
Yield: ½ cup
Prep time: 5 minutes
Cook time: none

To vary the flavor of this versatile vinaigrette, add fresh herbs such as thyme or chives, or substitute chopped shallots for the garlic. Serve on green salads, or sprinkled over grilled or roasted chicken or fish.

2 tablespoons fresh lemon juice

1 medium clove garlic, minced

½ teaspoon kosher salt

½ teaspoon freshly ground black pepper

6 tablespoons extra-virgin olive oil

In a small bowl, combine the lemon juice, garlic, salt, and pepper. Slowly whisk in the extra-virgin olive oil until the dressing is slightly thickened. Alternatively, place all ingredients in a jar with a tight-fitting lid and shake until well combined.

Nutritional Analysis

Per 2-tablespoon serving: 190 Calories, 21 g Fat, 2.9 g Sat, 0 mg Chol,

0 g Fiber, 0 g Protein, 0 g Carb, 240 mg Sodium

Pomegranate Vinaigrette

Phase I: Detox
Gluten Free
Dairy Free
Quick
Vegetarian
Egg Free

Serves 5
Serving size: 2 tablespoons
Yield: about ⅔ cup
Prep time: 5 minutes
Cook time: none

Red in color and subtle in flavor, this vinaigrette is especially good with bitter salad greens such as escarole, frisée, arugula, or radicchio. Pomegranate molasses is a thick, dark syrup made from the juice of pomegranates. It adds a tart, sharp yet sweet flavor to the marinade and is available from specialty markets, some larger supermarkets, and Internet retailers.

3 tablespoons pomegranate juice

1 tablespoon fresh lemon juice

1 teaspoon pomegranate molasses

½ teaspoon minced garlic (about 1 small clove)

½ teaspoon Dijon mustard

½ teaspoon kosher salt

½ teaspoon freshly ground black pepper

6 tablespoons extra-virgin olive oil

In a medium bowl, mix together the pomegranate juice, lemon juice, pomegranate molasses, garlic, mustard, salt, and pepper. Slowly whisk in the extra-virgin olive oil until the dressing is slightly thickened. Alternatively, place all ingredients in a jar with a tight-fitting lid and shake until well combined.

Nutritional Analysis

Per 2-tablespoon serving: 169 Calories, 17 g Fat, 2.4 g Sat, 0 mg Chol,

0 g Fiber, 0 g Protein, 4 g Carb, 206 mg Sodium

Lime-Rice Wine Vinaigrette

A tart, sweet vinaigrette, especially good on a salad served with Asian food.

2 teaspoons fresh lime juice

2 teaspoons unseasoned rice wine vinegar

½ teaspoon kosher salt

¼ teaspoon white pepper

¼ cup extra-virgin olive oil

Phase I: Detox
Gluten Free
Dairy Free
Quick
Vegetarian
Egg Free

Serves 4
Serving size: 2 tablespoons
Yield: about ½ cup dressing
Prep time: 5 minutes
Cook time: none

In a small bowl, combine the lime juice, vinegar, salt, and pepper. Slowly whisk in the extra-virgin olive oil until the dressing is slightly thickened. Alternatively, place all ingredients in a jar with a tight-fitting lid and shake until well combined.

Nutritional Analysis

Per 2-tablespoon serving: 129 Calories, 14 g Fat, 2.0 g Sat, 0 mg Chol,

0 g Fiber, 0 g Protein, 1 g Carb, 263 mg Sodium

Mustard Vinaigrette

Phase I: Detox
Gluten Free
Dairy Free
Quick
Vegetarian
Egg Free

Serves 4
Serving size: 2 tablespoons
Yield: ½ cup
Prep time: 5 minutes
Cook time: none

A versatile vinaigrette, this can be used on any green salad, or with potato salad.

2 tablespoons fresh lemon juice
2 teaspoons whole-grain mustard
1 teaspoon minced garlic
½ teaspoon kosher salt
½ teaspoon freshly ground black pepper
6 tablespoons extra-virgin olive oil

In a small bowl, combine the lemon juice, mustard, garlic, salt, and pepper. Slowly whisk in the extra-virgin olive oil until the dressing is slightly thickened. Alternatively, place all ingredients in a jar with a tight-fitting lid and shake until well combined.

Nutritional Analysis

Per 2-tablespoon serving: 195 Calories, 21 g Fat, 2.9 g Sat, 0 mg Chol,

0 g Fiber, 1 g Protein, 1 g Carb, 300 mg Sodium

Pistachio Basil Pesto

Rich and delicious, this dairy-free pesto is the perfect complement to grilled chicken, fish, or cooked whole grains. If the pesto is too thick, add a small quantity of vegetable broth or hot water to thin it. Easy to make ahead, it freezes beautifully in any small, tightly covered freezer container.

8 ounces shelled pistachios

4 ounces pine nuts

1 cup moderately packed basil

2 medium cloves garlic, chopped

¾ cup extra-virgin olive oil

½ teaspoon kosher salt

¼ teaspoon freshly ground black pepper

Preheat the oven to 350 degrees F.

Place the pistachios and pine nuts on a rimmed baking sheet and toast in the oven for 6 to 7 minutes, until lightly browned. Remove to a plate to cool.

Combine the pistachios, pine nuts, basil, garlic, extra-virgin olive oil, salt, and pepper in the bowl of a food processor fitted with a metal blade and process until smooth.

To freeze pesto: Pour the pesto into ice-cube trays. Freeze until solid. Remove the pesto cubes from the trays and store in a zip-top bag. Thaw and use the pesto as needed.

Nutritional Analysis

Per 2-tablespoons serving: 222 Calories, 22 g Fat, 2.6 g Sat, 0 mg Chol,

2 g Fiber, 4 g Protein, 6 g Carb, 60 mg Sodium

Phase I: Detox
Gluten Free
Dairy Free
Quick
Vegetarian
Egg Free

Serve 16
Serving size: 2 tablespoons
Yield: 2 cups
Prep time: 15 minutes
Cook time: none

Phase I

Vinaigrettes, Sauces, and Dressings

Spicy Cilantro-Lime Vinaigrette

Phase I: Detox
Gluten Free
Dairy Free
Quick
Vegetarian
Egg Free

Serves 5
Serving size: 2 tablespoons
Yield: about ⅔ cup
Prep time: 10 minutes
Cook time: none

With the fresh flavor of lime juice, this vinaigrette pairs well with Romaine and Avocado Salad with Toasted Pumpkin Seeds (page 87).

3 tablespoons minced cilantro

3 tablespoons fresh lime juice

1 teaspoon minced garlic (about 1 medium clove)

¼ teaspoon kosher salt

¼ teaspoon ground chipotle pepper

¼ teaspoon freshly ground black pepper

6 tablespoons extra-virgin olive oil

In a small bowl, combine the cilantro, lime juice, garlic, salt, ground chipotle pepper, and black pepper. Slowly whisk in the extra-virgin olive oil until the dressing is slightly thickened. Alternatively, place all ingredients in a jar with a tight-fitting lid and shake until well combined.

Nutritional Analysis

Per 2-tablespoon serving: 200 Calories, 22 g Fat, 3.1 g Sat, 0 mg Chol,

0 g Fiber, 0 g Protein, 0.5 g Carb, 195 mg Sodium

Chicken Satay with Peanut Sauce

Easily made ahead and grilled before serving, these tasty hors d'oeuvres make a nice addition to an appetizer buffet. The peanut sauce is a little spicy, but kids would love the plain, marinated grilled chicken.

Phase II: Maintenance
Gluten Free
Dairy Free
Egg Free

Serves 16
Serving size: 3 pieces
Yield: 48 pieces
Prep time: 20 minutes
Cook time: 20 minutes

Chicken Satay

1½ pounds boneless, skinless chicken breasts, sliced into 3 x 1-inch strips
¾ cup canned unsweetened lite coconut milk
3 tablespoons low-sodium wheat-free tamari
1½ teaspoons Thai Kitchen Red Chili Paste
1½ teaspoons honey
1½ tablespoons chopped cilantro, plus ¼ cup for garnish
½ teaspoon kosher salt

Peanut Sauce

½ cup water
½ cup smooth natural peanut butter
2 teaspoons honey
1 teaspoon Thai Kitchen Red Chili Paste
1 teaspoon low-sodium wheat-free tamari
¼ teaspoon ground coriander
¼ teaspoon ground cumin
½ cup canned unsweetened lite coconut milk
3 tablespoons fresh lime juice

Soak 48 (8-inch) wooden skewers in water for 30 minutes.

To prepare the chicken, place the chicken strips in a shallow dish. Mix together the coconut milk, tamari, red chili paste, honey, cilantro, and salt. Pour over the chicken and refrigerate for 30 to 60 minutes.

Meanwhile, to make the sauce, mix together the water, peanut butter, honey, red chili paste, salt, tamari, coriander, and cumin in a small saucepan over low heat. Stir until the ingredients are well combined. Add the coconut milk and cook over low heat for 5 minutes, stirring frequently. Stir in the lime juice.

After the chicken has marinated, thread it lengthwise onto the skewers, using 1 strip of chicken per skewer. Heat an outdoor grill, or a stovetop grill pan lightly brushed with extra-virgin olive oil, to medium high. Grill the chicken for about

2 minutes. Turn and continue to cook for 1 more minute, until done. Lay the finished skewers on a platter, and sprinkle with the chopped cilantro. Serve with the peanut sauce on the side.

Nutritional Analysis

Per 3-piece serving: 102 Calories, 4.2 g Fat, 3.3 g Sat, 25 mg Chol,

1 g Fiber, 12 g Protein, 3 g Carb, 135 mg Sodium

Curried Deviled Eggs with Cashews

The addition of curry powder and chopped cashews gives this classic egg dish a new twist.

Phase II: Maintenance
Gluten Free
Dairy Free
Quick
Vegetarian

Serves 4
Serving size: 2 halves
Yield: 8 halves
Prep time: 30 minutes
Cook time: none

4 hard-boiled eggs, peeled and sliced in half

2 tablespoons Homemade Mayonnaise (page 258) or organic soy mayonnaise

¾ teaspoon curry powder

½ teaspoon rice wine vinegar

½ teaspoon agave nectar

¼ teaspoon grated fresh ginger

Pinch kosher salt

Pinch of freshly ground black pepper

1 tablespoon minced scallions

8 large raw, unsalted cashews, finely chopped

Remove the yolks from the eggs and place in a small bowl. Add the mayonnaise, curry powder, vinegar, agave nectar, ginger, salt, and pepper and mash with a fork. Stir in the minced scallions.

With a small spoon or melon baller, place an equal amount of the yolk mixture into each egg-white half. Sprinkle with the chopped cashews. Serve immediately, or cover with plastic wrap and refrigerate.

Nutritional Analysis

Per 2 halves: 173 Calories, 14 g Fat, 3.3 g Sat, 220 mg Chol, 0 g Fiber, 7 g Protein, 5 g Carb, 159 mg Sodium

Eggplant Caponata

A classic blend of Mediterranean flavors. The flavors intensify when served a day after making the caponata. Serve as part of an antipasto platter, or fill tricolored pepper wedges with this delightful mixture.

Phase II: Maintenance
Gluten Free
Dairy Free
Vegetarian
Egg Free

Serves 12
Serving size: ¼ cup
Yield: 3 cups
Prep time: 30 minutes
Cook time: 45 minutes

1 large eggplant (about 1 to 1¼ pounds), cut into 1-inch cubes

2 teaspoons kosher salt

1¼ cups extra-virgin olive oil

3 large celery ribs, cut into ½-inch dice (about 1 cup)

1 medium red onion, cut into ½-inch dice (about 1 cup)

8 ounces canned low-sodium whole tomatoes, drained and coarsely chopped

1 tablespoon low-sodium tomato paste

2 tablespoons water

8 to 10 pitted Kalamata olives, chopped (about ¼ cup)

4 to 6 pitted green Sicilian olives, chopped (about ¼ cup)

3 tablespoons red wine vinegar

1 tablespoon drained capers

1 teaspoon honey

Place the eggplant cubes in a colander over a bowl, and sprinkle with 1 teaspoon of the salt. Place a plate on the eggplant, and then place a heavy can on the plate to press down the eggplant. Let the eggplant rest for about 1 hour to extract any bitter juice.

Heat ¼ cup of the extra-virgin olive oil over medium heat in a heavy saucepan. Add the celery and cook for 5 minutes. Add the onion and the remaining 1 teaspoon salt and cook for 5 minutes. Add the tomatoes, tomato paste, and water, and cook for 10 minutes. Add the olives, red wine vinegar, capers, and honey, and cook for 5 minutes. Remove from the heat and set aside.

When the eggplant has drained, rinse briefly under cold water and pat dry with paper towels. Heat the remaining 1 cup of extra-virgin olive oil in a medium skillet over medium-high heat. Add the eggplant in batches and cook, stirring, until golden brown. Remove and drain on paper towels. Stir the cooked eggplant into the tomatoes and vegetables. Stir and place over medium heat. Simmer for about 5 minutes before serving.

Nutritional Analysis

Per ¼-cup serving: 123 Calories, 11 g Fat, 1.5 g Sat, 0 mg Chol, 2 g Fiber, 1 g Protein, 6 g Carb, 312 mg Sodium

Endive Spears with Middle Eastern Yogurt Dip

Phase II: Maintenance
Gluten Free
Quick
Vegetarian
Egg Free

Serves 4
Serving size: ¼ cup
Yield: 1 cup dip
Prep time: 15 minutes
Cook time: none

A tangy and somewhat spicy dip with a taste of mint. Aleppo pepper is a Turkish chile, with an ancho chile–like flavor, but perhaps a little hotter and more tart. If Aleppo pepper is not available, substitute crushed red pepper flakes or freshly ground black pepper to taste. Greek yogurt is thick because it's strained, and is similar to sour cream in texture.

1 cup nonfat Greek yogurt

2 tablespoons extra-virgin olive oil

¼ teaspoon kosher salt

¼ teaspoon Aleppo pepper

2 tablespoons fresh lemon juice

2 tablespoons minced mint

1 teaspoon minced garlic

2 tablespoons extra-virgin olive oil (optional)

4 medium heads Belgian endive, separated into individual leaves

Stir together the yogurt, extra-virgin olive oil, salt, Aleppo pepper, lemon juice, mint, and garlic.

Drizzle with the additional extra-virgin olive oil if desired, and serve with the endive leaves.

Nutritional Analysis

Per ¼-cup serving: 108 Calories, 7 g Fat, 1.0 g Sat, 1 mg Chol, 4 g Fiber, 4 g Protein, 10 g Carb, 156 mg Sodium

Salmon Spread with Lemon Mayonnaise

Serve this quick, elegant hors d'oeuvre at room temperature for the best flavor and ease of spreading. Serve with raw vegetables and fresh apple wedges. If you don't want to make the mayonnaise, use an organic store-bought soy mayonnaise.

2 cups chopped cooked or canned wild salmon (about 12 ounces)

2 tablespoons chopped dill

3 tablespoons snipped chives

2 tablespoons minced red onion

½ cup Homemade Mayonnaise (page 258), or ½ cup organic soy mayonnaise

2 tablespoons plus 1 teaspoon fresh lemon juice

1 teaspoon whole-grain mustard

½ teaspoon kosher salt

½ teaspoon freshly ground black pepper

Phase II: Maintenance
Gluten Free
Dairy Free
Quick
Egg Free (with soy mayonnaise)

Serves 6
Serving size: ¼ cup
Yield: 1½ cups
Prep time: 20 minutes
Cook time: none

In a medium bowl, combine the salmon, dill, chives, and onion. Add the mayonnaise, lemon juice, mustard, salt, and pepper. Stir well to combine.

Nutritional Analysis

Per ¼-cup serving: 234 Calories, 19 g Fat, 2.8 g Sat, 55 mg Chol,

0 g Fiber, 15 g Protein, 1 g Carb, 298 mg Sodium

Raspberry Yogurt Smoothie

Phase II: Maintenance
Gluten Free
Dairy Free
Quick
Vegetarian
Egg Free

Serves 2
Serving size: 1 (6-ounce)
smoothie
Yield: 2 (6-ounce)
smoothies
Prep time: 10 minutes
Cook time: none

You can also serve this for breakfast with a handful of granola.

1¼ cups frozen raspberries (5 ounces)

6 ounces plain nonfat soy yogurt

2 tablespoons water

2 tablespoons 100% freshly squeezed orange juice

Combine the raspberries, yogurt, water, and orange juice in a blender. Blend until smooth.

Nutritional Analysis

Per 6-ounce serving: 100 Calories, 1 g Fat, 0.6 g Sat, 6 mg Chol, 6 g Fiber, 6 g Protein, 19 g Carb, 72 mg Sodium

Strawberry Tofu Smoothie

Phase II: Maintenance
Gluten Free
Dairy Free
Quick
Vegetarian
Egg Free

Serves 2
Serving size: 1 (8-ounce)
smoothie
Yield: 2 (8-ounce)
smoothies
Prep time: 10 minutes
Cook time: none

Vanilla extract is the secret ingredient for enhancing the flavor of this creamy smoothie.

1¼ cups frozen strawberries (about 5 ounces)

1 cup silken soft tofu (8 ounces)

¼ cup cold water

4 tablespoons 100% freshly squeezed orange juice

¼ teaspoon vanilla extract

Combine all ingredients in a blender. Blend until smooth. Pour into glasses and serve.

Nutritional Analysis

Per 8-ounce serving: 122 Calories, 3 g Fat, 0.4 g Sat, 0 mg Chol, 2 g Fiber, 8 g Protein, 15 g Carb, 44 mg Sodium

Anytime Snack Mix

A quick and delicious snack. Serve as an afternoon snack for the kids, or for adults to munch on with a glass of sparkling water with pomegranate juice.

¼ cup raw, unsalted cashews

¼ cup raw, unsalted pecan halves

¼ cup raw, unsalted whole almonds

¼ cup raw, unsalted walnuts pieces

¼ cup hulled raw, unsalted sunflower seeds

6 tablespoons dried organic cranberries

6 tablespoons organic golden raisins

Preheat the oven to 400 degrees F.

Mix together the cashews, pecans, almonds, walnuts, and sunflower seeds on a baking sheet. Bake for 5 minutes. Cool the nut mixture slightly. Mix in the dried cranberries and raisins. Store in tightly covered glass bowls.

Phase II: Maintenance
Gluten Free
Dairy Free
Quick
Vegetarian
Egg Free

Serves 6
Serving size: generous
¼ cup
Yield: 1¾ cups
Prep time: 5 minutes
Cook time: 5 minutes

Nutritional Analysis

Per ¼-cup serving: 213 Calories, 15 g Fat, 1.6 g Sat, 0 mg Chol,

2.5 g Fiber, 5 g Protein, 20 g Carb, 4 mg Sodium

Honey-Roasted Spiced Pecans

Phase II: Maintenance
Gluten Free
Dairy Free
Vegetarian
Egg Free

Serves 6
2 heaping tablespoons
Yield: 1 cup
Prep time: 5 minutes
Cook time: 1 hour and
15 minutes

These nuts are slightly sweet, spicy, and salty. A good snack and easy to make, it needs to dry in the oven for almost an hour, so plan accordingly.

¾ teaspoon ground cumin

½ teaspoon crushed red pepper flakes

½ teaspoon kosher salt

¼ teaspoon ground coriander

1 tablespoon honey

1 tablespoon grapeseed oil

1 cup pecan halves

Preheat the oven to 250 degrees F. Line a baking sheet with parchment paper.

Mix together the cumin, red pepper flakes, salt, and coriander.

Heat the honey and grapeseed oil in a medium skillet over medium heat until the honey dissolves. Add the pecans, and stir to coat the nuts evenly with the honey. Cook over low heat for about 3 minutes. Add the spices and cook for 3 minutes.

Turn the pecan mixture onto the baking sheet. Bake for about 45 minutes. Remove the parchment paper and place the pecans directly on the sheet pan. Separate the nuts, if desired, so they do not clump together. Bake for 30 minutes, until the pecans are dry to the touch. Stir the pecans occasionally while baking.

Let the pecans cool, and store in an airtight container.

Nutritional Analysis

Per 2-heaping-tablespoon serving: 157 Calories, 15 g Fat, 3 g Sat, 0 mg Chol,

2 g Fiber, 2 g Protein, 8 g Carb, 161 mg Sodium

UltraMetabolism Road Mix

Cocoa nibs are roasted cocoa beans separated from their husks and broken into small bits. The nibs can be used in recipes or as a stand-alone snack when nothing but chocolate will satisfy your taste buds.

½ cup dried wild blueberries

1 cup cocoa nibs

1 cup raw almonds, whole

1 cup raw cashews, whole

1 cup raw walnuts, whole

1 cup hulled raw pumpkin seeds

1 cup hulled raw sunflower seeds

In a medium bowl, mix all the ingredients. Store in a covered jar and keep in a cool, dark place.

Nutritional Analysis

Per ½-cup serving: 300 Calories, 24 g Fat, 0 mg Chol, 10 g Fiber, 13 g Protein, 23 g Carb, 54 mg Sodium

Phase II: Maintenance

Gluten Free

Dairy Free

Quick

Vegetarian

Egg Free

Serves 13

Serving size: ½ cup

Yield: 6½ cups

Prep time: 5 minutes

Cook time: none

Baked Fruit

Phase II: Maintenance
Gluten Free
Dairy Free
Quick
Vegetarian
Egg Free

Serves 3
Serving size: 1⅓ cups
Yield: 4 cups
Prep time: 10 minutes
Cook time: 15 minutes

Fresh fruit in season, such as apples, pears, peaches, plums, and apricots

1 tablespoon balsamic vinegar

¼ teaspoon ground cardamom

Preheat the oven to 375 degrees F.

Cut the fruit into 1- to 2-inch cubes. You'll need 4 cups of cubes. Place in a shallow baking dish. Drizzle with the balsamic vinegar and sprinkle with the cardamom. Bake for 15 minutes or until fruit is tender.

Nutritional Analysis

Per 1-cup serving: 150 Calories, 0 g Fat, 0 g Sat, 0 g Chol, 4 g Fiber, 2 g Protein, 30 g Carb, 0 g Sodium

Butternut Squash Bisque

This vegetable bisque is satisfying, smooth, and slightly spicy.

3 tablespoons extra-virgin olive oil

1 medium clove garlic, finely chopped (about 1 teaspoon)

1 tablespoon finely diced ginger

½ cup chopped leek, white and pale green parts only

½ cup diced celery

½ cup diced carrot

1 large butternut squash (about 3 pounds), peeled and diced

½ teaspoon kosher salt

½ teaspoon freshly ground black pepper

4 cups organic chicken or vegetable stock or broth

1 cup shelled raw, unsalted pumpkin seeds

2 tablespoons low-sodium wheat-free tamari

1 teaspoon honey

¼ teaspoon ground cinnamon

⅛ teaspoon ground nutmeg

¼ cup finely snipped chives

Phase II: Maintenance
Gluten Free
Dairy Free
Vegetarian (with vegetable
stock or broth)
Egg Free

Serves 10
Serving size: 1 cup
Yield: 10 cups
Prep time: 40 minutes
Cook time: 35 minutes

Heat the extra-virgin olive oil in a large soup pot over medium heat. Add the garlic, ginger, leek, celery, and carrot. Cook for about 10 minutes, until the leek and celery start to soften. Add the squash, salt, and pepper and cook for 10 minutes. Stir in the chicken or vegetable stock or broth. Bring the soup to a boil, then reduce the heat to a simmer. Cook for 15 minutes, or until all the vegetables are tender enough to pierce with a fork.

Meanwhile, toast the pumpkin seeds in a small skillet over medium heat for about 3 to 4 minutes. Stir the pumpkin seeds frequently and watch closely to prevent burning. When toasted, remove the seeds to a plate.

When the soup is finished cooking, remove it from the heat and let cool slightly. Purée the soup in batches in a blender, returning the batches to a large saucepan. Stir in the tamari, honey, cinnamon, and nutmeg. Heat the soup through.

Serve garnished with the snipped chives and toasted pumpkin seeds.

Nutritional Analysis

Per 1-cup serving: 183 Calories, 11 g Fat, 2.0 g Sat, 10 mg Chol,

4 g Fiber, 7 g Protein, 17 g Carb, 381 mg Sodium

Dilled Egg Salad on Baby Spinach

A wonderful way to enjoy more omega-3 fats.

Phase II: Maintenance
Gluten Free

Serves 2
Serving size: 2 cups
Yield: 4 cups
Prep time: 15 minutes
Cook time: 20 minutes

4 whole omega-3 eggs

2 tablespoons finely chopped scallions

2 tablespoons finely chopped fresh dill

2 tablespoons organic soy mayonnaise

2 teaspoons Dijon mustard

Pinch kosher salt

Dash freshly ground black pepper

3 cups fresh baby spinach, trimmed and washed

1 large red apple, cut into wedges

Place the eggs in a medium saucepan and cover with cold water. Bring to a boil over medium-high heat. Remove from the heat, cover, and let stand for 15 minutes. Drain the eggs and plunge them into ice water to chill. When cold, peel and coarsely chop.

Combine the eggs, scallions, dill, mayonnaise, mustard, salt, and pepper in a medium bowl and toss gently. Arrange the spinach and apple wedges on a salad plate, and top with the egg salad.

Nutritional Analysis

Per 2-cup serving: 270 Calories, 15 g Fat, 3.6 Sat, 423 mg Chol,

4 g Fiber, 15 g Protein, 19 g Carb, 398 mg Sodium

Baby Arugula, Shaved Fennel, and Cranberry Salad with Hazelnut Vinaigrette

Phase II: Maintenance
Gluten Free
Dairy Free
Quick
Vegetarian
Egg Free

Serves 6
Serving size: 1½ cups
Yield: 9 cups
Prep time: 10 minutes plus
15 minutes to make the
vinaigrette
Cook time: none

A pretty salad with a delicious combination of spicy arugula, shaved fennel, and the tart, sweet taste of dried cranberries. The hazelnut vinaigrette with chopped toasted hazelnuts adds even more interesting flavor and texture. To prepare the fennel, use a sharp vegetable peeler and shave very thin slices off the bulb.

8 cups baby arugula, washed and dried (about 4 ounces)

1 cup shaved fennel (about 2 ounces)

½ cup dried cranberries

1 recipe Hazelnut Vinaigrette (page 257)

12 chives, cut into 2-inch lengths

In a salad bowl, combine the arugula, fennel, and cranberries. Add the vinaigrette and toss to combine.

Garnish with the chive pieces.

Nutritional Analysis

Per 1½-cup serving: 174 Calories, 14 g Fat, 1.0 g Sat, 0 mg Chol,

2 g Fiber, 2 g Protein, 12 g Carb, 258 mg Sodium

Phase II: Maintenance
Gluten Free
Dairy Free
Quick
Vegetarian
Egg Free

Serves 4
Serving size: 2 cups
Yield: 8 cups
Prep time: 20 minutes
Cook time: none

Frisée, Escarole, and Blood Orange Salad with Orange–White Wine Vinaigrette

Raspberry-red blood oranges and pomegranate seeds are a colorful complement to the greens. For the prettiest salad, leave the frisée leaves whole.

2 medium blood oranges

¼ cup slivered blanched almonds (about 1 ounce)

4 cups frisée leaves, washed and dried

4 cups escarole hearts, washed, dried, and torn into bite-size pieces

¼ cup thinly sliced red onion

¼ cup pomegranate seeds

1 recipe Orange–White Wine Vinaigrette (page 260)

Cut the peel and white membrane off the oranges with a sharp knife. Gently remove the sections, cutting in between the membranes.

Toast the almonds in a small skillet over medium-low heat for about 3 to 5 minutes. Stir the almonds frequently and watch closely to prevent burning. When toasted, remove the almonds to a plate to cool.

In a large salad bowl, combine the frisée, escarole, orange sections, toasted almonds, onion slices, and pomegranate seeds. Drizzle ½ cup of the vinaigrette over the salad. Gently toss to mix. Serve immediately.

Nutritional Analysis

Per 2-cup serving: 240 Calories, 18 g Fat, 2.3 g Sat, 0 mg Chol,

6 g Fiber, 4 g Protein, 18 g Carb, 363 mg Sodium

Herb Salad

This salad is best with the freshest herbs available and makes a great accompaniment to grilled fish, poultry, or lean meat. Mesclun, or a mix of young, assorted salad greens, provides the base for the salad.

½ cup chopped raw, unsalted walnuts

½ cup tarragon leaves

½ cup small basil leaves

½ cup small mint leaves

4 cups mesclun or assorted baby salad greens

½ cup parsley leaves

Phase II: Maintenance
Gluten Free
Dairy Free
Quick
Vegetarian
Egg Free

Serves 4
Serving size: 1¾ cups
Yield: 7 cups
Prep time: 15 minutes
Cook time: none

½ cup fresh dill, stems removed

½ cup chives, cut in 2-inch lengths

½ recipe Sherry-Walnut Vinaigrette (page 251)

Toast the walnuts in a small skillet over medium–low heat for 5 to 6 minutes, until lightly colored. Transfer to a plate to cool.

Gently tear the tarragon, basil, and mint leaves into small pieces if the leaves are large; otherwise, combine the mesclun, whole herb leaves, and chives in a medium bowl. Add the toasted walnuts, and toss with the vinaigrette.

Nutritional Analysis

Per 1¾-cup serving: 245 Calories, 24 g Fat, 2.4 g Sat, 0 mg Chol,

3 g Fiber, 4 g Protein, 7 g Carb, 208 mg Sodium

Edamame, Tomato, and Green Bean Salad with Sesame Dressing

Phase II: Maintenance
Gluten Free
Dairy Free
Quick
Vegetarian
Egg Free

Serves 6
Serving size: 1 cup
Yield: 6 cups
Prep time: 30 minutes
Cook time: none

Slender green beans work perfectly in this salad, contrasting with the textures of the edamame and tomato. Sesame dressing adds flavor, and the black sesame seeds add crunch. If black seeds are unavailable, white or brown sesame seeds may be substituted.

1 (14-ounce) package frozen shelled edamame

12 ounces whole thin green beans, stem ends trimmed

5 ounces grape tomatoes, halved (about 1 cup)

2 tablespoons black sesame seeds

4 tablespoons sesame oil

2 tablespoons rice wine vinegar

1 tablespoon low-sodium wheat-free tamari

2 teaspoons honey

½ teaspoon kosher salt

Bring a large pan of salted water to a boil. Drop in the edamame and cook for about 3 to 4 minutes, until tender but still firm. Using a sieve, remove the edamame from the water and immediately place them in a bowl of ice water to stop the cooking. Drain and shake dry. Place in a large bowl.

Return the water to a boil and add the green beans. Cook until crisp-tender, about 1 to 2 minutes. Drain, and immediately place in a bowl of ice water to cool. Drain and pat dry. Add to the edamame, along with the halved tomatoes.

Toast the sesame seeds in a small skillet over medium-low heat for about 5 minutes. Remove to a plate to cool.

To make the dressing, in a small bowl, mix together the sesame oil, rice wine vinegar, tamari, honey, and salt. Pour over the vegetables and sprinkle with the toasted sesame seeds.

Nutritional Analysis

Per 1-cup serving: 213 Calories, 13 g Fat, 1.4 g Sat, 0 mg Chol, 6 g Fiber, 8.5 g Protein, 15 g Carb, 229 mg Sodium

Napa Cabbage Slaw

Crisp and lemony, this refreshing salad contains a colorful mix of vegetables.

Phase II: Maintenance
Gluten Free
Dairy Free
Quick
Vegetarian
Egg Free

Serves 6
Serving size: generous
¾ cup
Yield: 4½ cups
Prep time: 30 minutes
Cook time: none

2 cups thinly sliced Napa cabbage

1 cup thinly sliced radicchio

1 cup julienne or matchstick carrot pieces

½ cup thinly sliced scallion (about 3 scallions)

¼ cup shredded daikon

2 tablespoons minced cilantro

1 tablespoon minced mint

¼ cup extra-virgin olive oil

2 tablespoons fresh lemon juice

2 tablespoons rice wine vinegar

1 teaspoon honey

½ teaspoon kosher salt

In a large bowl, combine the cabbage, radicchio, carrot, scallion, daikon, cilantro, and mint.

In a medium bowl, whisk together the extra-virgin olive oil, lemon juice, rice wine vinegar, honey, and salt. Pour the dressing over the vegetables and mix well.

Nutritional Analysis

Per ¾-cup serving: 140 Calories, 12 g Fat, 1.6 g Sat, 0 mg Chol, 2 g Fiber, 1 g Protein, 8 g Carb, 216 mg Sodium

Roasted Beet Salad with Warm Goat Cheese

Phase II: Maintenance
Gluten Free
Vegetarian
Egg Free

Serves 4
Serving size: 1 cup
Prep time: 35 minutes
Cook time: 50 to 60 minutes

The citrus vinaigrette brings out the sweetness of the beets and is a nice contrast to the slightly bitter frisée. The warm goat cheese is creamy and smooth, with a slight hint of thyme. Kalamata or Gaeta olives work best for this dish, a great first course or a main-course lunch.

4 medium beets, stem and root ends trimmed

½ cup pecans

4 (1-ounce) round slices soft goat cheese, such as Montrachet

1 tablespoon extra-virgin olive oil

Pinch of kosher salt

¼ teaspoon coarsely ground black pepper

⅛ teaspoon chopped thyme

1 small bunch frisée (about ¼ pound), trimmed, washed, and dried (4 cups)

1 recipe Citrus Vinaigrette (page 254)

12 brine-cured black olives, pitted and halved

1 tablespoon snipped chives

Preheat the oven to 450 degrees F.

Wrap the beets in a double layer of aluminum foil. Place the beets in the oven and roast for 50 to 60 minutes, until tender when pierced with a knife. Remove them from the oven and allow to cool. When the beets are cool, rub them with paper towels to remove the skins. Cut the beets into ½-inch cubes. They can be prepared a few days ahead and refrigerated.

Meanwhile, toast the pecans in a small skillet over medium heat for about 4 to 5 minutes, until slightly darker in color. Stir frequently and watch closely to prevent burning. When toasted, remove the nuts to a plate to cool.

Place the cheese rounds on a glass pie plate. Brush the cheese on both sides with the extra-virgin olive oil. Sprinkle with the salt, pepper, and thyme. Refrigerate until ready to use.

When ready to assemble the salad, preheat the oven to 400 degrees F.

Bake the goat cheese rounds for 3 to 4 minutes, until just warmed but not melted. Remove from the oven.

To assemble the salad, toss the beets and the frisée, separately, with ¼ cup of the vinaigrette. Divide the beets among 4 plates. Divide the frisée into 4 portions and arrange on the plates with the beets. Place 1 round of warm goat cheese on each plate and garnish with the toasted pecans, olives, and snipped chives. Drizzle with the remaining vinaigrette if desired.

Nutritional Analysis

Per 1-cup serving: 341 Calories, 29 g Fat, 6.7 g Sat, 13 mg Chol,

4 g Fiber, 9 g Protein, 14 g Carb, 479 mg Sodium

Quinoa and Arugula Salad with Balsamic Dressing

The nutty texture of quinoa pairs nicely with tender arugula and herbs.

Phase II: Maintenance
Dairy Free
Quick
Vegetarian
Egg Free

Serves 4
Serving size: ¾ cup
Yield: 3 cups
Prep time: 15 minutes
Cook time: 20 minutes

2 cups water

½ teaspoon kosher salt

1 cup quinoa, rinsed

¼ cup balsamic vinegar

1 medium clove garlic, crushed with the back of a knife

¼ teaspoon freshly ground black pepper

¼ cup extra-virgin olive oil

3 cups baby arugula, washed and dried

½ cup grape tomatoes, cut in half (about 6 ounces)

¼ cup thinly sliced red onion

2 tablespoons chopped parsley

2 tablespoons thinly sliced basil

Bring the water and ¼ teaspoon of the salt to a boil in a medium saucepan. Add the quinoa and cook, covered, at a gentle simmer for 15 to 17 minutes, until the quinoa is tender but firm and the water has been absorbed. Put the quinoa in a large bowl and let cool to room temperature.

Meanwhile, in a medium bowl, whisk together the balsamic vinegar, garlic, the remaining ¼ teaspoon salt, and the pepper. Slowly whisk in the extra-virgin olive oil until the dressing is slightly thickened. Remove the garlic clove.

In a salad bowl, combine ¼ cup of the balsamic dressing and the quinoa. Add the arugula, tomatoes, onion, parsley, and basil, and stir gently to mix. Add more dressing if desired.

Nutritional Analysis

Per ¾-cup serving: 309 Calories, 17 g Fat, 2.0 g Sat, 0 mg Chol, 3 g Fiber, 7 g Protein, 34 g Carb, 262 mg Sodium

Wild Salmon Salad Niçoise

This beautiful, tasty remake of traditional Salad Niçoise uses roasted salmon instead of tuna. A perfect light supper or lunch, you can serve it in half portions for a nice first course.

Phase II: Maintenance
Gluten Free
Dairy Free

Serves 4 as a main course
or 8 as an appetizer
Prep time: 40 minutes
Cook time: 20 minutes

- 8 small red potatoes (about 1½ ounces each)
- 8 ounces whole thin green beans, stem ends trimmed
- 4 (5-ounce) wild salmon fillets
- 7 tablespoons extra-virgin olive oil
- 2 tablespoons fresh lemon juice
- 1½ teaspoons freshly ground black pepper
- 2 tablespoons red wine vinegar
- 2 medium cloves garlic
- 1 teaspoon Dijon mustard
- 3 anchovy fillets
- 1 teaspoon kosher salt
- 24 grape or cherry tomatoes, halved
- 8 cups mixed tender salad greens
- 4 hard-boiled eggs, peeled and cut in half
- 24 Niçoise olives
- 2 tablespoons finely snipped chives

Place the potatoes in a medium pan. Cover the potatoes with cold water. Bring to a boil and cook for about 10 to 12 minutes, until the potatoes are tender when pierced with a small knife. Drain and set aside. When cool enough to handle, cut the potatoes into quarters.

Bring a small pan of water to a boil. Add the green beans and cook for about 1 minute, until crisp-tender. Drain and immediately place in a bowl of ice water to cool. Drain and set aside.

Preheat the oven to 450 degrees F.

Place the salmon in a shallow baking dish and coat with 1 tablespoon of the extra-virgin olive oil, the lemon juice, ½ teaspoon of the salt, and the pepper. Bake for about 12 minutes, or until the salmon has reached desired doneness.

Combine the red wine vinegar, garlic, mustard, anchovies, the remaining 6 tablespoons of extra-virgin olive oil, salt, and the remaining 1 teaspoon pepper in the bowl of a small food processor fitted with a metal blade or in a blender, and process until smooth.

To assemble the salad:

Coat the potatoes, green beans, and tomatoes with dressing, using 1½ tablespoons of dressing for the potatoes, 1½ tablespoons for the green beans, and 1 tablespoon for the tomatoes. In a large bowl, toss the salad greens with 3 tablespoons of dressing.

Divide the salad greens among 4 (or 8) plates. Decoratively place the salmon, potatoes, green beans, tomatoes, eggs, and olives on the plate. Sprinkle with the snipped chives.

Nutritional Analysis

Per main-course serving: 644 Calories, 40 g Fat, 7.2 g Sat, 281 mg Chol,

7 g Fiber, 43 g Protein, 28 g Carb, 480 mg Sodium

Phase II: Maintenance
Gluten Free
Vegetarian
Egg Free

Serves 4
Serving size: 2½ cups
greens plus ½ pear
Yield: 10 cups salad
greens plus 2 pears
Prep time: 25 minutes
Cook time: 35 minutes

Winter Salad with Pears, Ricotta Salata, and Lemon-Mustard Vinaigrette

Use greens such as frisée, radicchio, escarole hearts, endive, or romaine hearts in this elegant, perfect-for-winter salad.

2 large firm Bosc pears, peeled, cored, and cut into 8 wedges

2 teaspoons extra-virgin olive oil

¼ teaspoon freshly ground black pepper

½ cup walnut halves

10 cups mixed salad greens, washed and dried

½ cup ricotta salata, crumbled into small pieces

1 recipe Lemon-Mustard Vinaigrette (page 249)

2 tablespoons finely snipped chives

Preheat the oven to 450 degrees F.

Place the pears in a single layer on a baking sheet. Drizzle with the extra-virgin olive oil and sprinkle with the pepper.

Place the pears in the oven and roast for about 15 minutes. Using tongs or a fork, turn the pears over on the baking sheet and roast for about 10 minutes more, until they begin to turn golden brown.

Meanwhile, toast the walnuts in a small skillet over medium-low heat, stirring for about 8 to 10 minutes, until lightly colored. When the nuts are toasted, remove to a plate.

In a large bowl, combine the greens with ½ cup of the vinaigrette and toss gently to coat. Add more vinaigrette to taste.

Divide the dressed salad greens onto 4 plates. Place 4 wedges of the roasted pears on each plate, next to the greens. Sprinkle with the crumbled cheese and toasted walnuts. Garnish with a sprinkle of chives.

Nutritional Analysis

Per 2½ cups greens plus ½ pear: 499 Calories, 44 g Fat, 8.0 g Sat, 13 mg Chol,

7 g Fiber, 7 g Protein, 24 g Carb, 517 mg Sodium

Crunchy Asian Peanut Salad

Phase II: Maintenance
Serves 2
Serving size: 2 cups
Yield: 4 cups
Prep time: 20 minutes
Cook time: none

A nutty, tangy salad you can eat anytime.

Peanut Miso Lime Dressing

¼ cup chunky style natural peanut butter

¼ cup extra-virgin olive oil

¼ cup dark miso paste

4 tablespoons freshly squeezed lime juice

¼ cup water

Salad

1 cup shredded Napa cabbage

1 cup julienned jicama

1 cup grated carrots

½ cup sliced almonds

½ fresh orange, cut into wedges

1 cup bean sprouts

1 cup edamame beans, thawed

Prepare the dressing by mixing all ingredients until well blended and smooth. Place all salad ingredients in a large mixing bowl. Pour dressing over the salad and toss until thoroughly mixed.

Nutritional Analysis

Per 2-cup serving: 398 Calories, 24 g Fat, 2.9 g Sat, 0 mg Chol,

11 g Fiber, 22 g Protein, 31 g Carb, 83 mg Sodium

Peanut Miso Lime Dressing: 125 Calories, 11 g Fat, 1.4 g Sat, 0 mg Chol,

1 g Fiber, 3 g Protein, 4 g Carb, 322 mg Sodium

Totals: 523 Calories, 35 g Fat, 4.3 g Sat, 0 mg Chol, 12 g Fiber, 25 g Protein, 35 g Carb, 405 mg Sodium

Apple-Soy Roasted Salmon

A moist and tasty salmon fillet with a spicy, sweet golden-brown glaze. A squeeze of lime juice finishes the dish.

¾ cup 100% apple juice

4 (6-ounce) wild salmon fillets

2 tablespoons low-sodium wheat-free tamari

1 tablespoon sesame oil

1 teaspoon agave nectar

1 teaspoon minced garlic

1 teaspoon minced ginger

¼ teaspoon Thai Kitchen Red Chili Paste

2 scallions, thinly sliced on the diagonal

4 lime wedges

Phase II: Maintenance
Gluten Free
Dairy Free
Egg Free

Serves 4
Serving size: 1 (6-ounce) fillet
Yield: 4 salmon fillets
Prep time: 15 minutes plus 1 hour marinating time
Cook time: 21 minutes

Place the apple juice in a small pan. Bring to a boil over high heat and reduce by about half. When reduced, set aside to cool.

Place the salmon in a single layer in a shallow baking dish.

Stir into the cooled, reduced apple juice, the tamari, sesame oil, agave nectar, garlic, ginger, and red chili paste. Pour the marinade over the salmon and refrigerate for about 1 hour.

Preheat the oven to 450 degrees F.

Before roasting the salmon, pour the excess marinade off the fish into a small pan. Bring the marinade to a boil over high heat. Cook until reduced by half, about 7 minutes.

Place the salmon in the oven and cook for about 7 minutes. Brush salmon with the reduced marinade and continue cooking for about 7 more minutes, or until golden brown and cooked through. Before serving, brush again with the marinade, and garnish with the scallions and lime wedges.

Nutritional Analysis

Per 6-ounce serving: 397 Calories, 23 g Fat, 5.0 g Sat, 123 mg Chol,

0 g Fiber, 38 g Protein, 8 g Carb, 270 mg Sodium

Balsamic-Glazed Fish Fillets

Phase II: Maintenance
Gluten Free
Dairy Free
Quick
Egg Free

Serves 4
Serving size: 6 ounces
Yield: 4 (6-ounce) fillets
Prep time: 10 minutes plus
marinating time
Cook time: 8 to 10 minutes

Balsamic marinade produces a nice crust on the outside of the fish. Cook over medium to medium-high heat, as high heat causes too much charring. The fish is best if marinated for 3 to 4 hours. Black cod, striped bass, or salmon are suggested for best results.

4 (6-ounce) skinless fish fillets, ¾ to 1 inch thick

¼ cup balsamic vinegar

¼ cup extra-virgin olive oil

2 medium cloves garlic, minced

2 teaspoons finely minced shallot

1 tablespoon finely chopped parsley

1 teaspoon finely chopped oregano

½ teaspoon kosher salt

½ teaspoon freshly ground black pepper

4 lemon wedges

2 tablespoons finely chopped herbs such as chives, oregano, parsley, or basil

Place the fish in a shallow dish. Combine the vinegar, extra-virgin olive oil, garlic, shallot, parsley, oregano, salt, and pepper. Pour over the fish, cover, and refrigerate for 2 to 4 hours, turning the fish at least once.

Preheat an outdoor grill or indoor grill pan brushed with olive oil over medium heat. Place the fish on the grill and cook for 5 minutes. Turn and continue cooking for 1 to 5 more minutes, until desired degree of doneness. The time will vary depending on the type of fish and the thickness of the fillets.

Serve with a squeeze of fresh lemon juice and a sprinkle of fresh herbs.

Nutritional Analysis

Per 6-ounce serving: 237 Calories, 11 g Fat, 1.8 g Sat, 140 mg Chol,

0 g Fiber, 31 g Protein, 1 g Carb, 122 mg Sodium

Citrus-Marinated Cod with Miso Dressing

This fish cooks crisp and brown on the outside and moist on the inside. The combination of fish, lime, scallion, and miso dressing is refreshingly delicious. This could also be prepared on an outdoor grill or under the broiler. If black cod, or sable, is not available, striped bass is a tasty substitute.

Phase II: Maintenance
Gluten Free
Dairy Free
Egg Free

Serves 4
Serving size: 1 (6-ounce)
fillet plus 2 tablespoons
dressing
Yield: 4 (6-ounce) fillets
Prep time: 10 minutes plus
1 hour marinating time
Cook time: 10 minutes

4 (6-ounce) black cod fillets

¼ cup 100% fresh-squeezed orange juice

3 tablespoons extra-virgin olive oil

1 tablespoon low-sodium wheat-free tamari

¼ teaspoon kosher salt

1 teaspoon freshly ground black pepper

1 recipe Miso Dressing (page 259)

1 lime, cut into 4 wedges

4 small thinly sliced scallions

Place the fish fillets in a shallow dish. Combine the orange juice, 2 tablespoons of extra-virgin olive oil, the tamari, salt, and pepper. Pour over the fillets and refrigerate for about 1 hour.

Preheat a grill pan brushed with the remaining 1 tablespoon extra-virgin olive oil until hot but not smoking. Remove the fillets from the marinade, shaking off the excess marinade. Place the fish in the pan and cook for 5 minutes. Turn and continue cooking for 4 to 5 minutes, until it reaches desired degree of doneness.

To serve, place 2 tablespoons of the miso dressing on each plate. Set the cooked fish on top of the dressing. Squeeze one lime wedge on each piece of fish and top with the sliced scallions.

Nutritional Analysis

Per 6-ounce fillet and 2 tablespoons dressing: 327 Calories, 22 g Fat,

3.1 g Sat, 65 mg Chol, 1 g Fiber, 28 g Protein, 5 g Carb, 489 mg Sodium

Miso-Marinated Fish Fillets

Phase II: Maintenance
Gluten Free
Dairy Free
Egg Free

Serves 6
Serving size: 1 (6-ounce) fillet
Yield: 6 (6-ounce) fillets
Prep time: 10 minutes plus 2 hours marinating time
Cook time: 18 minutes

The miso marinade gives the fish a delicate taste. Marinate the fish for two hours for best results. Longer marinating time will produce a more intense flavor, and the depth of flavor depends on the thickness of the fish. Also, for a thicker piece of fish, adjust the cooking time accordingly.

6 (6-ounce) fish fillets, such as striped bass or cod

3 tablespoons light gluten-free miso

3 tablespoons low-sodium wheat-free tamari

3 tablespoons rice wine vinegar

1 tablespoon honey

½ teaspoon Thai Kitchen Red Chili Paste

1 teaspoon grated fresh ginger

6 lime wedges

Place the fish in a shallow baking dish.

In a small bowl, whisk together the miso, tamari, vinegar, honey, red chili paste, and ginger, until smooth. Pour the marinade over the fish. Cover and refrigerate for about 2 hours.

Preheat the oven to 400 degrees F.

Pour off and reserve excess marinade. Bake the fish for about 18 minutes for a fillet that is ¾ inch thick. Cooking time will vary with the thickness of the fish. Brush the fish with the marinade during cooking. Serve with the lime wedges.

Nutritional Analysis

Per 6-ounce serving: 202 Calories, 5 g Fat, 0.9 g Sat, 140 mg Chol,

0 g Fiber, 32 g Protein, 6 g Carb, 804 mg Sodium

Wild Salmon Cakes with Asian Cabbage Slaw

Hijiki is a type of sea vegetable that tastes similar to Japanese nori, the sea vegetable that is most often used in sushi. It is loaded with minerals, including iodine, which helps the thyroid function, and adds a wonderful, fresh flavor to this dish.

Phase II: Maintenance
Gluten Free
Dairy Free

Serves 2
Serving Size: 3 patties,
2 cups salad
Yield: 6 patties,
4 cups salad
Prep time: 20 minutes
Cook time: 10 minutes

6 ounces canned wild salmon, chopped fine

½ cup diced red pepper

¼ cup diced scallions

½ cup diced celery

¼ cup soy flour

2 tablespoons minced cilantro

1 whole omega 3-type egg

pinch kosher salt

dash freshly ground black pepper

1 tablespoon sesame oil

2 cups shredded Napa cabbage

2 cups seedless cucumbers, sliced very thin (skin on)

1 cup daikon radish, sliced very thin

¼ cup hijiki, soaked

¼ cup plain unseasoned rice vinegar

2 tablespoons honey

2 tablespoons chopped cilantro

In a large mixing bowl, add the salmon, peppers, scallions, celery, soy flour, cilantro, egg, salt, and pepper. Mix together well and form into six patties. Preheat a medium skillet over medium-high heat. Add sesame oil and swirl pan to coat evenly. Add patties and cook for 3–5 minutes on each side. Meanwhile, toss together the cabbage, cucumbers, daikon radish, hijiki, rice vinegar, honey and cilantro in a large bowl. Divide salad between two serving plates. Place salmon cakes on top of salad. Serve.

Nutritional Analysis

Per 3 patties and 2 cups Slaw: 406 Calories, 16 g Fat, 3 g Sat, 126 mg Chol,

5 g Fiber, 31 g Protein, 41 g Carb, 221 mg Sodium

Pan-Seared Scallops with Peach Kiwi Salsa, Baby Bok Choy, and Steamed Kasha

Phase II: Maintenance
Dairy Free
Egg Free

Serves 2
Serving size: 2 cups
scallops, 2 baby bok choy
with kasha
Prep time: 20 minutes
Cook time: 10 minutes

Getting the scallops nice and brown on the outside adds a wonderful dimension to the flavor and texture of this dish. The addition of fruit and honey make for a slightly sweet flavor that is very complementary. Kiwis are rich in fiber, potassium, and vitamin C and are a nutrient-dense addition to salads, salsas, and chutneys.

1 tablespoon extra-virgin olive oil

1 pound fresh sea scallops, patted dry

½ cup minced red onion

1 cup frozen peaches, defrosted and diced small

3 peeled and diced kiwi

1 teaspoon honey

1 teaspoon freshly squeezed lime juice

Apple-Soy Roasted Salmon (page 203)

Turkey and Red Bean Chili (page 114)

Seafood Salad with Lemon Dressing (page 126)

Vegetable Omelet with Manchego Cheese (page 246)

Seafood Salad with Lemon Dressing (page 126)

Vegetable Omelet with Manchego Cheese (page 246)

Chicken Cacciatore (page 116)

Pork Tenderloin with Mojo Sauce (page 210)

Super Bowl Sunday Dip (page 70)
and Grilled Shrimp Brochettes
(page 97)

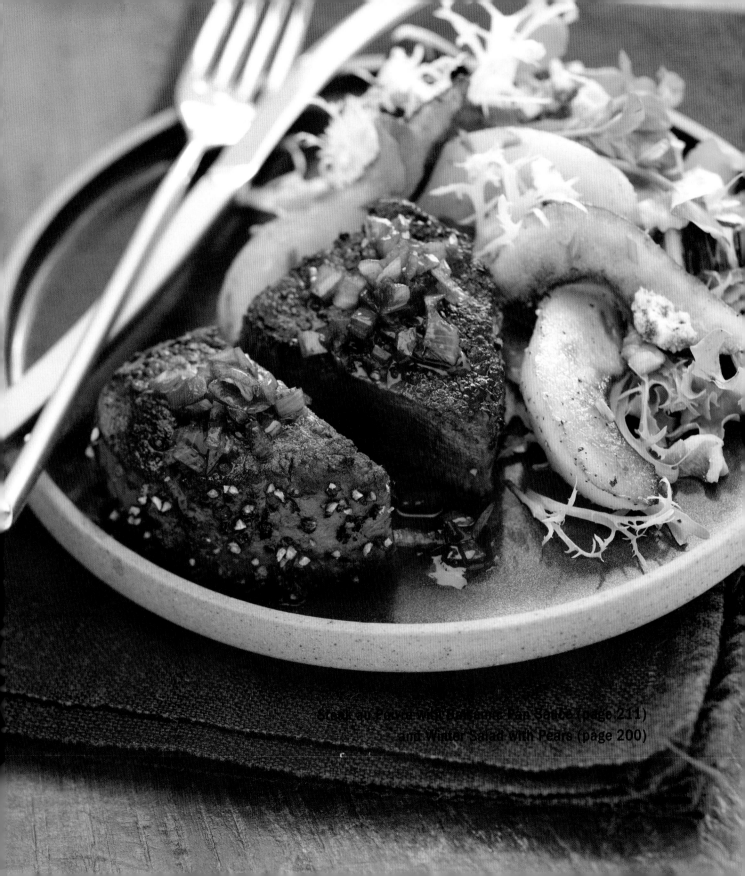

Steak au Poivre with Balsamic Pan Sauce (page 211)
and Winter Salad with Pears (page 200)

pinch of kosher salt
¼ cup washed and chopped cilantro

4 heads baby bok choy
1 cup buckwheat groats (kasha), steamed

Heat a medium-size skillet over medium heat until hot. Add extra-virgin olive oil and swirl pan to evenly distribute. Add the scallops one at a time in a single layer. Let scallops cook undisturbed for 2 to 3 minutes until scallops are nice and brown on the bottom. Carefully turn scallops over and cook on the other side for 3 more minutes. Remove pan from heat and let scallops sit in the pan while you prepare the salsa.

Combine the onion, peaches, kiwi, honey, lime juice, salt, and cilantro in a medium size bowl. Mix well.

Meanwhile, steam baby bok choy. Place cooked kasha and scallops on top of the bok choy with a spoonful of the salsa.

Nutritional Analysis

Per 2 cups scallops and 2 baby bok choy with kasha: 549 Calories, 12 g Fat, 0 g Sat, 60 mg Chol,

13 g Fiber, 43 g Protein, 62 g Carb, 903 mg Sodium

Pork Tenderloin with Mojo Sauce

Phase II: Maintenance
Gluten Free
Dairy Free
Egg Free

Here is a tasty and tender meat to grill in summertime, perfect served with fresh corn and sliced tomatoes. If desired, the mojo sauce can be made one day ahead of time and stored in the refrigerator until used.

Serves 6
Serving size: 4 ounces
Yield: 1½ pounds
Prep time: 15 minutes
Cook time: 15 to 20 minutes

2 (about ¾ pound each) whole pork tenderloins, trimmed

3 tablespoons extra-virgin olive oil

1 tablespoon plus 2 teaspoons minced garlic

½ teaspoon kosher salt

½ teaspoon freshly ground black pepper

½ cup 100% fresh-squeezed orange juice

2 tablespoons fresh lime juice

2 tablespoons minced cilantro

2 teaspoons minced oregano

1 teaspoon minced jalapeño pepper

½ teaspoon ground cumin

Rub the pork with 1 tablespoon of extra-virgin olive oil, 2 teaspoons of the garlic, ¼ teaspoon of the salt, and the black pepper. Cover and refrigerate for at least 1 hour, or overnight.

In a small bowl, mix together the orange juice, lime juice, cilantro, oregano, jalapeño pepper, cumin, the remaining ¼ teaspoon salt, the remaining extra-virgin olive oil, and the remaining 1 tablespoon of chopped garlic.

Preheat an outdoor grill to medium-high or brush an indoor grill pan lightly with olive oil, and heat over high heat until hot but not smoking. Alternatively, preheat the oven to 450 degrees F.

Grill the meat for about 8 minutes. Turn and cook for 7 to 9 more minutes to cook evenly. Alternatively, roast in the oven for about 20 minutes.

Let the meat rest for 10 minutes before slicing. Serve drizzled with the mojo sauce.

Nutritional Analysis

Per 4-ounce serving: 208 Calories, 11 g Fat, 2.3 g Sat, 63 mg Chol,

0 g Fiber, 23 g Protein, 3 g Carb, 206 mg Sodium

Steak au Poivre with Balsamic Pan Sauce

An elegant, special-occasion entrée. The filet mignon is extremely tender, and the mustard and peppercorns produce nice crusts. The balsamic vinegar reduction adds a deep color and flavor.

Phase II: Maintenance
Gluten Free
Dairy Free
Egg Free

Serves 4
Serving size: 1 (6-ounce) steak
Yield: 4 (6-ounce) steaks
Prep time: 15 minutes
Cook time: 20 minutes

1 tablespoon black peppercorns, coarsely ground or cracked

2 teaspoons green peppercorns, coarsely ground or cracked

1 teaspoon pink peppercorns, coarsely ground or cracked

4 (6-ounce) filet mignon steaks

1 tablespoon Dijon mustard

1 teaspoon kosher salt

3 tablespoons extra-virgin olive oil

¼ cup minced shallots

½ cup balsamic vinegar

Mix the black, green, and pink peppercorns together on a large plate.

Pat the steaks dry with a paper towel. Brush the steaks with the mustard. Roll in the peppercorns and sprinkle with the salt. Press down on the steaks so that the peppercorns adhere to the meat.

Heat the extra-virgin olive oil in a skillet, large enough to hold the steaks, over medium-high heat. Add the steaks and cook for 5 minutes. Turn and cook for 5 more minutes for medium-rare, or until desired degree of doneness is reached.

Cooking time will vary with the thickness of the meat. Remove the steaks to a plate when finished cooking.

Reduce the heat to medium and add the shallots to the skillet. Cook, stirring, about 3 to 4 minutes, until softened. Add the balsamic vinegar, turn up the heat to medium-high, and cook, scraping up any brown bits from the bottom of the skillet, until the vinegar is slightly thickened and syrupy. Drizzle the sauce over the steaks and serve.

Nutritional Analysis

Per 6-ounce serving: 323 Calories, 17 g Fat, 3.8 g Sat, 90 mg Chol,

1 g Fiber, 34 g Protein, 11 g Carb, 623 mg Sodium

Thai-Style Beef and Vegetable Curry

Phase II: Maintenance
Gluten Free
Dairy Free
Egg Free

Serves 4
Serving size: 2 cups
Yield: 8 cups
Prep time: 25 minutes
Cook time: 15 minutes

A tasty one-dish meal that can be prepared in less than an hour. For those who like their curry hot, increase the red chili paste to 2 teaspoons.

4 ounces thin green beans, stem ends trimmed

1 cup broccoli florets

1¼ cups canned unsweetened lite coconut milk

1 teaspoon Thai Kitchen Red Chili Paste

2 tablespoons raw, unsalted cashews, chopped

2 tablespoons light sesame oil

2 tablespoons dark sesame oil

1 medium red bell pepper, cored, seeded, and cut into ¾-inch pieces (about 1 cup)

2 large shiitake mushrooms, stems removed and caps cut into ¼-inch strips

½ cup julienne carrot

½ teaspoon kosher salt

1 pound beef sirloin, trimmed and cut crosswise into thin strips

½ cup thinly sliced basil

1 tablespoon fresh lime juice

Lime wedges

Bring a large pot of salted water to a boil. Drop the beans into the water and cook for about 1 minute, until crisp-tender. With a sieve, scoop out the beans and place in a bowl of ice water to stop the cooking. Return the water to a boil. Drop in the broccoli and cook for about 30 seconds, until crisp-tender. Drain and place the broccoli in the ice water to stop the cooking. Drain the broccoli and set aside.

In a small bowl, stir together the coconut milk and red curry paste. Set aside.

Toast the cashews in a small skillet over medium heat for 3 to 4 minutes, until lightly colored. Remove to a plate to cool.

Heat 1 tablespoon of the light sesame oil and 1 tablespoon of the dark sesame oil in a large skillet over medium-high heat. Add the red pepper and cook, stirring, for 30 seconds. Add the mushrooms and cook, stirring, for 2 minutes. Add the green beans, broccoli, carrot, and ¼ teaspoon salt and cook, stirring, for 1 minute. Transfer the vegetables to a bowl.

Heat the remaining 1 tablespoon light and 1 tablespoon dark sesame oil in the same skillet. Add the beef and cook on one side for about 2 minutes. Sprinkle with ¼ teaspoon salt. Turn and cook on the other side until browned. Add the coconut milk mixture. Bring to a boil and cook for about 3 minutes, until slightly reduced. Stir in the cooked vegetables and heat through. Add the basil and lime juice.

Serve garnished with the toasted cashews and lime wedges.

Nutritional Analysis

Per 2-cup serving: 401 Calories, 28.25 g Fat, 3.25 g Sat, 55 mg Chol,

4 g Fiber, 24 g Protein, 16 g Carb, 212 mg Sodium

Chicken Cutlets with Cornmeal Crust and Cilantro Buttermilk Dressing

A gluten-free alternative to traditional breaded chicken cutlets, these are crunchy on the outside, with the taste of toasted corn. Once the cutlets are prepared, they can be cooked immediately or refrigerated for up to two hours before cooking. They're good with a squeeze of lime juice, or even better served on top of fresh salad greens as a main-course salad, drizzled with the Cilantro Buttermilk Dressing (page 252).

Serves 4
Serving size: 1 chicken cutlet plus 2 tablespoons dressing
Yield: 4 chicken cutlets plus ½ cup dressing
Prep time: 10 minutes
Cook time: 3 minutes per batch

¼ cup chickpea or soy flour

¼ teaspoon kosher salt

¼ teaspoon freshly ground black pepper

1 large egg

1 teaspoon water

½ cup organic yellow cornmeal

1 pound boneless, skinless chicken breasts, pounded ¼-inch thick

3 tablespoons extra-virgin olive oil

Kosher salt (optional)

Lime wedges

1 recipe Cilantro Buttermilk Dressing (page 252)

On a large, flat plate, mix the flour with the salt and pepper. In a shallow bowl, beat the egg with the water. Place the cornmeal on a flat plate.

Dredge each chicken cutlet in the seasoned flour, shaking off the excess. Dip the chicken in the egg wash, coating evenly. Let the excess egg drip off. Then coat the chicken with the cornmeal. Place the cutlets on a rack until ready to cook.

Heat 2 tablespoons of the olive oil in a large skillet over medium–high heat until hot but not smoking. The oil is ready when the edge of the chicken sizzles when placed in the skillet. Cook the cutlets in batches, if necessary, for 1 to 2 minutes on each side, until golden and crisp. Do not overcrowd the pan. Add the remaining olive oil if necessary.

Sprinkle with coarse kosher salt if desired. Serve with lime wedges and Cilantro Buttermilk Dressing.

Nutritional Analysis

Per 1 cutlet plus 2 tablespoons dressing: 293 Calories, 13 g Fat, 2.8 g Sat,

124 mg Chol, 1 g Fiber, 30 g Protein, 9 g Carb, 249 mg Sodium

Grilled Chicken "Under a Brick"

This recipe may sound gimmicky, but chicken pressed and cooked under a brick is beautifully browned, crisp on the outside and succulent and juicy on the inside. Two bricks, individually wrapped in aluminum foil, make the best heavy weight for pressing the chicken.

Phase II: Maintenance
Gluten Free
Dairy Free
Egg Free

Serves 4
Serving size: ¼ chicken
Yield: 1 (3- to 3½-pound) chicken
Prep time: 15 minutes plus 1 hour marinating time
Cook time: 40 minutes

1 (3- to 3½-pound) whole chicken, backbone removed and flattened

3 tablespoons extra-virgin olive oil

2 tablespoons fresh lemon juice

2 teaspoons minced garlic (about 2 medium cloves)

2 teaspoons chopped thyme

2 teaspoons chopped rosemary

1 teaspoon crushed red pepper flakes

1½ teaspoon kosher salt

Lemon wedges for garnish

Place the chicken in a shallow dish.

In a small bowl, combine the extra-virgin olive oil, lemon juice, garlic, thyme, rosemary, red pepper flakes, and salt. Pour the marinade over the chicken. Cover and refrigerate for at least 1 hour, or overnight, turning the chicken in the marinade at least once. Longer marinating will produce more intense flavor.

Heat an outdoor grill, indoor grill pan, or a large cast-iron skillet to medium-high.

Remove the chicken from the marinade. Place it on the grill or in the pan, skin side down. Weight the chicken down with a heavy weight, such as two bricks wrapped in aluminum foil placed on a baking sheet. Cook over medium heat for 20 minutes. Turn the chicken and continue to cook for about 20 more minutes, until the outside is brown and crisp and an instant-read thermometer inserted in the thickest part of the chicken reads 170 degrees F.

Remove from the grill and cover loosely with foil. Allow the chicken to rest for 10 to 15 minutes. Cut the chicken into pieces and serve with lemon wedges.

Nutritional Analysis

Per ¼ chicken: 558 Calories, 38 g Fat, 9.1 g Sat, 196 mg Chol,

0 g Fiber, 50 g Protein, 1 g Carb, 388 mg Sodium

Stir-Fried Chicken and Broccoli with Cashews

Phase II: Maintenance
Gluten Free
Dairy Free
Egg Free

Serves 4
Serving size: 2 cups
Yield: 8 cups
Prep time: 30 minutes
(plus 30 minutes
marinating time)
Cook time: 12 minutes

A classic combination of chicken and broccoli, somewhat spicy from the red chili paste. Preserve the beautiful green color of the broccoli by first blanching it, as described below, and then stir-frying.

1¼ pounds boneless, skinless chicken breast, cut into ¼-inch-thick strips

6 tablespoons low-sodium wheat-free tamari

2 tablespoons rice wine vinegar

1 tablespoon dark sesame oil

1 teaspoon honey

1 teaspoon Thai Kitchen Red Chili Paste

1 medium head broccoli, cut into florets

½ cup raw, unsalted cashews, roughly chopped

2 teaspoons arrowroot

3 tablespoons light sesame oil

1 tablespoon minced garlic

2 teaspoons minced ginger

½ cup sliced scallion

2 cups steamed brown rice

Place the strips of chicken breast in a large bowl.

In a small bowl, combine the tamari, rice wine vinegar, honey, dark sesame oil, and red chili paste. Pour over the chicken. Cover and refrigerate for 30 minutes, or up to 2 hours.

Meanwhile, bring a large pot of salted water to a boil. Drop in the broccoli and cook for 1 minute. Drain, and place in a bowl of ice water to stop the cooking. Drain the broccoli and pat dry with paper towels. Set aside.

Toast the cashews in a small skillet over medium-low heat for 4 to 5 minutes, turning frequently, until lightly colored. When toasted, remove the nuts to a plate to cool.

Pour the excess marinade off the chicken into a small bowl. Stir in the arrowroot and set aside.

Heat the light sesame oil in a large skillet or wok over high heat. Add the chicken and cook, stirring quickly and constantly, for 2 minutes. Transfer to a plate.

Add the garlic and ginger and cook, stirring quickly and constantly, for 30 seconds. Add the broccoli and chicken and cook, stirring quickly and constantly, for about 2 minutes or until the chicken is cooked through. Add the scallions and the marinade. Cook for about 1 minute, until thickened. Add the toasted cashews and stir to combine and heat through.

Transfer to a platter and serve with the steamed brown rice.

Nutritional Analysis

Per 2-cup serving: 523 Calories, 25 g Fat, 4.3 g Sat, 82 mg Chol,

6 g Fiber, 42 g Protein, 34.5 g Carb, 1,066 mg Sodium

Shiitake Chinese Chicken with Brown Rice

Phase II: Maintenance
Dairy Free
Quick
Egg Free

Serves: 4
Prep Time: 20 minutes
Cook Time: 45 minutes

Chinese 5-spice seasoning is a standard stock pantry item in my kitchen that adds a sweet flavor to recipes. It is a blend of fennel, anise, ginger, licorice root, cloves, and cinnamon, spices that deliver valuable phytochemicals.

Sauce

2 tablespoons low-sodium wheat-free tamari

2 tablespoons mirin

1 cup low-sodium organic chicken broth

2 teaspoons arrowroot

⅛ teaspoon Chinese 5-spice seasoning

Chicken

4 scallions, sliced diagonally

2 cloves fresh garlic, pressed

1 tablespoon extra-virgin olive oil

2 tablespoons grated fresh ginger

1 pound skinless, boneless chicken tenders

2 large carrots, peeled and sliced diagonally

2 cups shiitake mushrooms

¼ pound snow peas, strings removed

2 cups chopped bok choy

2 cups steamed brown rice

To make the sauce: In a small bowl, whisk together the tamari, mirin, chicken broth, arrowroot, and seasoning.

Saute the scallions and garlic for 3 minutes in the olive oil in a wok or sauté pan over medium heat. Add ginger and chicken and continue to stir fry for another

2–3 minutes. Toss in the carrots, mushrooms, snow peas, and bok choy and stir for another 3 minutes. Add the sauce, cover, and cook for approximately 5 minutes. Serve over cooked brown rice.

Nutritional Analysis

Per serving: 409 Calories, 7 g Fat, 1 g Sat, 76 mg Chol, 7 g Fiber, 36 g Protein, 50 g Carb, 249 mg Sodium

Balsamic-Marinated Tofu with Herbs and Sautéed Spinach

Phase II: Maintenance
Gluten Free
Dairy Free
Vegetarian
Egg Free

Serves 4
Serving size: 1 slice tofu
plus ½ cup spinach
Yield: 4 slices tofu plus
2 cups spinach
Prep time: 10 minutes plus
1 hour or more to press,
drain, and marinate
Cook time: 6 minutes

This tofu with a Mediterranean flavor profile cooks to a beautiful brown color, with crispy edges. Allow time to press and drain the tofu before cooking.

1 (14-ounce) package extra-firm tofu

4 tablespoons extra-virgin olive oil

2 tablespoons balsamic vinegar

1 teaspoon minced garlic

1 teaspoon minced parsley

1 teaspoon minced rosemary

1 teaspoon minced thyme

¼ teaspoon kosher salt

½ teaspoon coarsely ground black pepper

1 recipe Sautéed Spinach with Garlic and Lemon (page 152)

Cut the tofu into 2 equal pieces. Slice each piece in half, horizontally, making a total of 4 slices. To press and drain the tofu, place the slices in a single layer on a shallow dish or tray, with paper towels underneath and on top of the tofu. Place another dish or tray on top of the tofu and weigh it down with several cans of food or a heavy skillet. Refrigerate for at least 30 minutes.

Meanwhile, combine 2 tablespoons of extra-virgin olive oil, the vinegar, garlic, parsley, rosemary, thyme, salt, and pepper.

After the tofu has drained, discard the excess liquid and pat the tofu dry with a paper towel. Place the tofu in a shallow dish and pour the balsamic marinade over it. Refrigerate for at least 30 minutes. Marinating longer will give the tofu a more intense flavor.

Heat the remaining extra-virgin olive oil over medium-high heat in a skillet large enough to hold the tofu in a single layer. Cook the tofu for 2 to 3 minutes

on each side, until brown and beginning to crisp. Remove to a plate when finished cooking.

Serve atop Sautéed Spinach with Garlic and Lemon.

Nutritional Analysis

Per 1 slice tofu and ½ cup spinach: 274 Calories, 23 g Fat, 3.3 g Sat, 0 mg Chol,

4 g Fiber, 12 g Protein, 9 g Carb, 615 mg Sodium

Vegetable-Tofu Stir-Fry

This colorful and delicious dish has a little heat on the finish and a subtle ginger flavor. Serve with steamed brown rice, if desired.

Phase II: Maintenance
Gluten Free
Dairy Free
Vegetarian
Egg Free

Serves 4
Serving size: 1 cup
Yield: 4 cups
Prep time: 25 minutes plus
30 minutes marinating
time
Cook time: 8 minutes

8 ounces extra-firm tofu, patted dry and cut into ¾-inch cubes

3 tablespoons low-sodium wheat-free tamari

1½ tablespoons rice wine vinegar

1½ teaspoons dark sesame oil

¾ teaspoon Thai Kitchen Red Chili Paste

2 teaspoons arrowroot

3 tablespoons light sesame oil

1 cup julienne carrots (about 2 ounces)

1 cup julienne daikon (about 3 ounces)

4 ounces shiitake mushrooms, stems removed,
    cut into ¼-inch slices (about 2 cups)

4 ounces snow peas, strings removed (about 1½ cups)

2 cups thinly sliced Napa cabbage (about 4 ounces)

2 cloves garlic, minced

1 teaspoon grated fresh ginger

¼ cup sliced scallions (about 2 medium)

1 tablespoon sesame seeds, toasted

Place the tofu in a shallow dish.

In a small bowl, whisk together the tamari, vinegar, dark sesame oil, and red chili paste. Pour over the tofu and turn the tofu to coat in the sauce. Cover and refrigerate for 30 minutes.

Drain and reserve the marinade. Whisk the arrowroot into the marinade.

Heat 1 tablespoon of the light sesame oil in a wok or large skillet over high heat. Add the tofu and cook, stirring quickly and constantly, for about 3 minutes, until brown. Transfer to a plate and reserve.

Heat the remaining 2 tablespoons light sesame oil. One at a time, add the carrots, daikon, mushrooms, snow peas, cabbage, garlic, and ginger, stir-frying each vegetable for about 30 seconds before adding the next vegetable. Stir the cooked tofu into the stir-fried vegetables. Add the reserved marinade and stir-fry for 1 minute to combine the flavors. Add the scallions. Serve sprinkled with the sesame seeds.

Nutritional Analysis

Per 1-cup serving: 241 Calories, 18 g Fat, 2.1 g Sat, 0 mg Chol,

3 g Fiber, 9 g Protein, 14.7 g Carb, 313 mg Sodium

Blackstrap Vegetarian Chili with Baby Greens Salad and Citrus Vinaigrette

Make a double batch of this easy chili, freeze in individual portions, and you will have it on hand for those extra-busy days.

Phase II: Maintenance
Gluten Free
Dairy Free
Vegetarian
Egg Free

Serves 4
Serving size: 1 cup
Yield: 4 cups
Prep time: 20 minutes
Cook time: 30 minutes

1 (15-ounce) can low-sodium kidney beans

1 (15-ounce) can low-sodium pinto beans

2 (14.5-ounce) cans low-sodium diced tomatoes with their juice

1 cup diced yellow onion

The UltraMetabolism Cookbook

½ cup chopped celery

2 tablespoons chopped fresh garlic

1 cup peeled, diced delicata squash

½ cup diced red bell pepper

2 cups low-sodium organic vegetable broth

2 tablespoons blackstrap molasses

3 tablespoons chili powder

1 tablespoon ground cumin

¼ cup extra-virgin olive oil

2 tablespoons freshly squeezed lemon juice

2 tablespoons balsamic vinegar

Pinch of kosher salt (optional)

Freshly ground pepper

Chopped fresh basil or other herb, to taste

2 teaspoons Dijon mustard

8 cups mixed baby greens

Combine the beans, tomatoes, onion, celery, garlic, squash, red pepper, broth, molasses, chili powder, and cumin in a large saucepan. Cover and simmer over medium-low heat for 20 minutes, until the vegetables are cooked through.

Whisk together the extra-virgin olive oil, lemon juice, balsamic vinegar, salt if desired, pepper, basil, and mustard. Pour over the greens in a large bowl and toss to coat. Serve the chili with the green salad.

Nutritional Analysis

Chili, per 1-cup serving: 381 Calories, 3 g Fat, .4 g Sat, 0 mg Chol,

24 g Fiber, 19 g Protein, 77 g Carb, 1060 mg Sodium

Salad, per 2-cup serving: 50 Calories, 0 g Fat, .9 g Sat, 0 mg Chol,

3 g Fiber, 3 g Protein, 10 g Carb, 69 mg Sodium

Citrus vinaigrette, per 1-tablespoon serving: 63 Calories, 7 g Fat, 1.2 g Sat, 0 mg Chol,

0 g Fiber, 0 g Protein, 1 g Carb, 14 mg Sodium

Grilled Portobello Mushrooms with Red Pepper Coulis

Phase II: Maintenance
Gluten Free
Vegetarian
Egg Free

Serves 2
Serving size: 1 mushroom,
plus 2½ tablespoons coulis
and 1 tablespoon goat
cheese
Yield: 2 mushrooms, plus
5 tablespoons coulis and
2 tablespoons goat cheese
Prep time: 20 minutes,
plus 1 hour marinating
time
Cook time: 10 minutes

In this satisfying vegetarian entrée, the mushrooms soak up the flavor of the marinade and are juicy after cooking. The red pepper coulis is a bit tangy, and pairs well with the goat cheese and basil garnish. If you want to roast your own red pepper, see page 150.

2 portobello mushrooms (about 6 ounces each)

3 tablespoons plus 1 teaspoons extra-virgin olive oil

2 tablespoons balsamic vinegar

1 teaspoon minced garlic

1 teaspoon minced flat-leaf parsley

½ teaspoon minced thyme

½ teaspoon minced rosemary

½ teaspoon kosher salt

¼ teaspoon freshly ground black pepper

½ cup roasted red pepper (about 1 medium pepper)

½ teaspoon champagne vinegar

Pinch of freshly ground black pepper

2 tablespoons soft goat cheese, such as Montrachet, for garnish

2 tablespoons thinly sliced basil, for garnish

Remove the stems from the mushrooms and wipe the tops clean with a damp paper towel. Using a small spoon, scrape out and discard the dark gills on the underside of the mushroom caps. Place the mushrooms on a cutting board or plate and press down to flatten.

In a small bowl, mix together 2 tablespoons plus 2 teaspoons of the extra-virgin olive oil, the vinegar, garlic, parsley, thyme, rosemary, ¼ teaspoon of the salt, and the pepper. Pour the mixture over the mushrooms, turning the mushrooms to coat. Let sit at room temperature for 1 hour.

Meanwhile, for the red pepper coulis, combine the roasted red pepper, the remaining extra-virgin olive oil, the champagne vinegar, the remaining ¼ teaspoon salt, and a pinch of pepper in the bowl of a food processor fitted with a metal blade. Process until smooth.

Just before cooking the mushrooms, heat a grill pan or a large skillet brushed with extra-virgin olive oil over medium-high heat. Cook the mushrooms until brown on both sides and tender when pierced with a knife, about 8 to 10 minutes.

To serve, cut each mushroom, on the diagonal, into 5 or 6 pieces. Fan the pieces on a plate and spoon about 2 tablespoons of the coulis over the top. Garnish with 1 tablespoon of the cheese and the basil.

Nutritional Analysis

Per mushroom plus 2½ tablespoons coulis and 1 tablespoon goat cheese: 331 Calories, 27 g Fat, 5.4 g Sat,

7 mg Chol, 4 g Fiber, 8 g Protein, 15 g Carb, 551 mg Sodium

Cranberry Pecan Wild Rice Salad

Phase II: Maintenance
Vegetarian
Dairy Free
Egg Free

Serves: 4
Prep time: 55 minutes
Cook time: none

Sage and turkey are classically complementary flavors. The cranberries in this salad add a delicious sweetness that nicely contrasts with the herby flavors.

Dressing

2 tablespoons walnut oil

1 tablespoon Dijon mustard

2 tablespoons apple cider vinegar

1 tablespoon chopped fresh sage

1 tablespoon chopped fresh thyme

Salad

⅔ cup cooked wild rice

½ cup grated carrots

2 tablespoons chopped red onion

6 ounces roast turkey breast, cubed

½ cup pecans

½ cup dried cranberries

Whisk together the oil, mustard, vinegar, sage, and thyme in a medium bowl. Add the carrots, onion, turkey, pecans, cranberries, and wild rice and toss gently. Serve.

Nutritional Analysis

Per serving: 380 Calories, 18 g Fat, 2 g Sat, 36 mg Chol, 5 g Fiber, 19 g Protein, 39 g Carb, 78 mg Sodium

Brown Basmati Rice Salad with Adzuki Beans

Phase II: Maintenance
Gluten Free
Dairy Free
Vegetarian
Egg Free

Serves 8
Serving size: ½ cup
Yield: 4 cups
Prep time: 25 minutes
Cook time: 35 to 40 minutes

A variation on classic red beans and rice, this should sit for a couple of hours to enhance the flavor. It should be made a few hours ahead of serving time and is a good accompaniment to food cooked on the grill during the summer.

4 tablespoons extra-virgin olive oil

3 tablespoons minced red onion

1 teaspoon minced garlic

1 cup brown basmati rice

1¾ cups water

½ teaspoon kosher salt

1 (15-ounce) can low-sodium adzuki beans, rinsed and drained

½ cup chopped celery

6 tablespoons finely chopped flat-leaf parsley

6 tablespoons thinly sliced scallions (about 6 medium scallions)

2½ teaspoons minced thyme

3 tablespoons red wine vinegar

¾ teaspoon freshly ground black pepper

Heat 1 tablespoon of extra-virgin olive oil in a small saucepan. Add the red onion and cook, stirring, for about 2 to 3 minutes, until translucent. Add the garlic and cook for 1 more minute. Stir in the rice to coat with the oil. Add the water and ¼ teaspoon of the salt. Bring to a boil, reduce the heat, cover, and simmer for about 35 minutes, until the water is absorbed and the rice is done.

Place the rice in a medium bowl. Add the beans, celery, parsley, scallions, and thyme.

Mix the vinegar, the remaining 3 tablespoons of extra-virgin olive oil, the remaining ¼ teaspoon salt, and the pepper. Pour ¼ cup of the dressing over the rice and mix. Add more dressing if desired. Serve at room temperature.

Nutritional Analysis

Per ½-cup serving: 195 Calories, 7.5 g Fat, 1.1 g Sat, 0 mg Chol, 4.5 g Fiber, 5 g Protein, 26 g Carb, 135 mg Sodium

Cranberry-Apricot Bulgur Salad

Phase II: Maintenance
Dairy Free
Quick
Vegetarian (with vegetable broth)
Egg Free

Serves 6
Serving size: ½ cup
Yield: 3 cups
Prep time: 20 minutes
Cook time: 10 minutes

A refreshing, colorful salad that is full of flavor, fruit, and crunch.

1 cup organic low-sodium chicken or vegetable broth

¼ cup water

1 teaspoon kosher salt

1 cup bulgur

¼ cup slivered blanched almonds

3 tablespoons extra-virgin olive oil

2 tablespoons fresh lemon juice

½ teaspoon freshly ground black pepper

⅓ cup dried cranberries

⅓ cup chopped unsulphured dried apricots

⅓ cup chopped flat-leaf parsley

2 tablespoons finely sliced scallions (about 2 small scallions)

In a small saucepan, combine the broth, water, and ½ teaspoon of the salt. Stir in the bulgur. Bring to a simmer, cover, and cook for about 5 to 6 minutes, until the liquid is absorbed. Remove from the heat and let the bulgur rest, covered, in the pan for 5 minutes.

Meanwhile, toast the almonds in a small skillet until golden brown, about 3 minutes. Remove to a plate to cool.

Pour the bulgur into a medium bowl and fluff it with a fork to remove any clumps.

Stir in the extra-virgin olive oil, lemon juice, pepper, and the remaining ½ teaspoon salt. Add the cranberries, apricots, parsley, and scallions. Stir well to combine.

Nutritional Analysis

Per ½-cup serving: 219 Calories, 10 g Fat, 1.3 g Sat, 1 mg Chol, 6 g Fiber, 5 g Protein, 30 g Carb, 355 mg Sodium

Quinoa Timbales with Roasted Pepper and Herbs

Baked in small ramekins, this unique and tasty side dish makes an attractive presentation. The roasted pepper and fresh herbs complement the quinoa.

Phase II: Maintenance
Gluten Free
Dairy Free
Vegetarian

Serves 6
Serving size: 4 ounces
Yield: 3 cups
Prep time: 30 minutes
Cook time: 50 minutes

1 cup quinoa (about 6 ounces)

2 cups water

½ teaspoon kosher salt

¼ cup pine nuts

2 tablespoons plus 2 teaspoons extra-virgin olive oil

½ cup minced onion

1 teaspoon minced garlic (about 1 medium clove)

1 large egg, lightly beaten

½ cup diced roasted red pepper (page 150)

¼ cup chopped basil

2 tablespoons minced flat-leaf parsley

1 teaspoon minced oregano

½ teaspoon freshly ground black pepper

6 teaspoons brown rice bread crumbs

Thoroughly rinse the quinoa in a fine-mesh strainer under cold running water until the water runs clear.

Bring the water to a boil in a 2-quart saucepan over high heat. Add the quinoa. Stir, reduce the heat to medium-low, cover, and simmer for about 12 minutes, until the water is absorbed. When the quinoa is done, remove it from the pan and place it in a medium bowl. Fluff with a fork to remove any lumps.

Meanwhile, toast the pine nuts in a small skillet and over medium-low heat for about 5 minutes, until they turn light golden brown. Stir frequently and watch closely to prevent burning. When toasted, remove the pine nuts to a plate to cool.

Heat 2 tablespoons of the extra-virgin olive oil in a medium skillet. Add the onion and ¼ teaspoon of salt and cook for about 3 minutes. Add the garlic and cook for about 3 minutes, until the onion and garlic are soft and translucent. Stir the cooked onion and garlic into the quinoa. Mix in the egg, red pepper, basil, parsley, oregano, the remaining ¼ teaspoon salt, and the black pepper.

Brush 6 (4-ounce) ramekins with the remaining 2 teaspoons of extra-virgin olive oil. Sprinkle each ramekin with 1 teaspoon of the brown rice bread crumbs and rotate to coat the bottom and sides with the bread crumbs. Shake out any excess.

Fill each ramekin with ½ cup of the quinoa mixture. Place the ramekins on a baking sheet and bake for about 25 minutes, until firm to the touch and beginning to brown around the edges. Remove from the oven, and let the timbales cool for 5 minutes. Place a small plate over the top of each ramekin, and invert the ramekins to remove the timbale. Carefully turn the timbales baked side up, and place them on a serving platter.

Nutritional Analysis

Per 4-ounce timbale: 266 Calories, 15 g Fat, 3.0 g Sat, 40 mg Chol,

2 g Fiber, 8 g Protein, 24 g Carb, 284 mg Sodium

Roasted Winter Vegetables with Raspberry Vinaigrette

Beautiful and delicious, these caramelized vegetables have flecks of fresh herbs throughout. The raspberry vinaigrette adds flavor and a glossy sheen to the dish.

12 ounces parsnips, peeled and cut into 1-inch pieces

12 ounces carrots, peeled and cut into 1-inch pieces

4 large cloves garlic, unpeeled

½ medium butternut squash, peeled and cut into 1-inch pieces

8 ounces (12 large) Brussels sprouts, trimmed and cut in half vertically

4 tablespoons extra-virgin olive oil

1 teaspoon minced rosemary

1 teaspoon minced thyme

1 teaspoon minced oregano

½ teaspoon kosher salt

½ teaspoon freshly ground black pepper

½ recipe Raspberry Vinaigrette (page 250)

Phase II: Maintenance
Gluten Free
Dairy Free
Vegetarian
Egg Free

Serves 6
Serving size: ⅔ cup
Yield: 4 cups
Prep time: 20 minutes
Cook time: 45 minutes

Preheat the oven to 425 degrees F.

In a large bowl, mix together the parsnips, carrots, garlic, butternut squash, Brussels sprouts, extra-virgin olive oil, rosemary, thyme, oregano, salt, and pepper. Toss well, coating the vegetables with extra-virgin olive oil, herbs, and seasonings.

Evenly divide the vegetables on 2 baking sheets. Place in the oven and roast for about 45 minutes, until the vegetables are soft and browned.

Transfer to a shallow bowl or platter. Squeeze the roasted cloves of garlic from their peels. Drizzle the raspberry vinaigrette over the vegetables, and serve.

Nutritional Analysis

Per ⅔-cup serving: 279 Calories, 19 g Fat, 2.7 g Sat, 0 mg Chol, 7 g Fiber, 3 g Protein, 27 g Carb, 302 mg Sodium

Cranberry-Apple Acorn Squash

Phase II: Maintenance
Gluten Free
Dairy Free
Vegetarian
Egg Free

Serves 4
Serving size: ½ of a
medium squash
Prep time: 15 minutes
Cook time: 1 hour

The tart yet sweet fruit and crunchy pecans give a real boost to the mild flavor of the squash. Easy to assemble, this dish needs an hour in the oven, but the results are worth the time!

2 teaspoons extra-virgin olive oil

2 medium acorn squash, thin slice removed from the top and bottom, then halved
   horizontally and seeds removed

½ cup dried cranberries

½ cup chopped, peeled apple

3 tablespoons 100% apple juice

3 tablespoons 100% cranberry juice

Pinch of kosher salt

Pinch of cinnamon

2 teaspoons water

½ teaspoon arrowroot

¼ cup chopped pecans

¼ teaspoon kosher salt

Pinch of freshly ground black pepper

Preheat the oven to 350 degrees F.

Brush a 13 x 9 x 2-inch baking dish with the extra-virgin olive oil. Place the squash, cut side down, in the dish and bake for 35 minutes.

Meanwhile, combine the cranberries, apples, apple juice, cranberry juice, pinch of salt, and pinch of cinnamon in a small saucepan over medium heat. Bring to a simmer and cook for 2 to 3 minutes, until the apples begin to soften.

In a small bowl, mix together the water and arrowroot. When the apples are soft, stir the arrowroot mixture into the apples and cranberries, bring to a gentle boil, and cook for 2 to 3 minutes, until the mixture is bubbling and thickened. Stir in the pecans.

When the squash has baked for 35 minutes, remove it from the oven. Flip the squash halves over, now with the cut side up. Sprinkle with salt and pepper and return to the oven. After 15 minutes, remove the squash from the oven and fill it with the cranberries and apples. Return the squash to the oven and bake for 15 minutes, or until soft.

Nutritional Analysis

Per ½ medium squash: 161 Calories, 3 g Fat, 0.4 g Sat, 0 mg Chol,

4 g Fiber, 2 g Protein, 37 g Carb, 250 mg Sodium

Green and Yellow Squash with Orange-Balsamic Dressing

A nice variation on roasted vegetables, this summer squash makes a delicious side dish with Pan-Browned Tilapia (page 98).

Phase II: Maintenance
Gluten Free
Dairy Free
Vegetarian
Egg Free

2 medium zucchini, cut into 1-inch cubes

2 medium yellow summer squash, cut into 1-inch cubes

3 tablespoons plus ½ teaspoon extra-virgin olive oil

½ teaspoon kosher salt

½ teaspoon freshly ground black pepper

1 head garlic, unpeeled, cut in half

1 tablespoon balsamic vinegar

1 teaspoon finely grated orange zest

Serves 4
Serving size: ½ cup
Yield: 2 cups
Prep time: 15 minutes
Cook time: 40 minutes

Preheat the oven to 425 degrees F.

Place the zucchini and summer squash on a large baking sheet. Toss with 2 tablespoons of the extra-virgin olive oil, the salt, and pepper.

Spread ½ teaspoon of the extra-virgin olive oil and a pinch of salt and pepper on the flat side of one of the garlic halves. Wrap it in aluminum foil and place on the baking sheet with the squash. Save the remaining piece of garlic for another use.

Place the squash and garlic in the oven and roast for about 40 minutes, until soft and beginning to brown. Turn once or twice while roasting.

While the squash is roasting, whisk together 1 tablespoon extra-virgin olive oil with the balsamic vinegar and orange zest.

Remove the squash from the oven and transfer to a serving platter. When cool enough to handle, squeeze the individual roasted garlic cloves from their skins and add them to the squash. Add half of the orange-balsamic mixture to the squash mixture and gently mix. Add more dressing if desired.

Nutritional Analysis

Per ½-cup serving: 152 Calories, 12 g Fat, 1.6 g Sat, 0 mg Chol,

2 g Fiber, 3 g Protein, 11 g Carb, 255 mg Sodium

Roasted Garlic and Shallots

Phase II: Maintenance
Gluten Free
Dairy Free
Vegetarian (with vegetable broth)
Egg Free

Serves 4
Serving size: 2 tablespoons
Yield: ½ cup
Prep time: 15 minutes
Cook time: 30 minutes

Use as a condiment for grilled or roasted meats as well as with a plain broiled or pan-fried steak. The garlic and shallots are soft and sweet from the slow cooking, and the balsamic vinegar adds dark, rich color and flavor.

12 medium cloves garlic, peeled

¼ cup plus 2 tablespoons extra-virgin olive oil

12 medium shallots, peeled

1 sprig of fresh thyme

½ cup organic low-sodium vegetable or chicken broth

1 teaspoon balsamic vinegar

Kosher salt

Freshly ground black pepper

1 tablespoon snipped chives

Preheat the oven to 425 degrees F.

Place the garlic in a small (6-inch) skillet or saucepan. Add ¼ cup of the extra-virgin olive oil and a pinch of salt and pepper. Cook over low heat, at a bare simmer, for 25 minutes, or until the garlic is soft and golden in color.

Mix the shallots, 1 tablespoon of extra-virgin olive oil, and a pinch of salt and pepper in a small ovenproof dish. Place the shallots in the oven and roast for 25 minutes, or until browned and soft.

After the garlic and shallots have both cooked, place the garlic and the remaining 1 tablespoon of extra-virgin olive oil from the garlic pan (save the remaining oil for another use) in another small saucepan. Add the roasted shallots and their oil, the thyme, and broth. Bring to a low boil, over medium heat, and cook for about 5 minutes, until the stock is reduced to about 1 tablespoon. Add the balsamic vinegar and cook for 30 to 60 seconds. Remove the thyme sprig and season to taste with salt and pepper. Garnish with the chives.

Nutritional Analysis

Per 2-tablespoon serving: 170 Calories, 11 g Fat, 1.6 g Sat, 3 mg Chol,

0 g Fiber, 4 g Protein, 17 g Carb, 18 mg Sodium

Amaranth with Orange-Berry Topping

Phase II: Maintenance
Gluten Free
Dairy Free
Vegetarian
Egg Free

Serves 4
Serving size: ¾ cup
plus 2 tablespoons
berry topping
Prep time: 10 minutes
Cook time: 25 minutes
Yield: 3 cups amaranth
plus ½ cup berry topping

The orange-berry topping makes the amaranth a delicious breakfast meal. The soy milk produces a thicker consistency than skim milk would and creates a dairy-free porridge.

1 cup amaranth
3 cups organic plain unsweetened soy milk
¼ teaspoon plus ⅛ teaspoon cinnamon
¼ teaspoon kosher salt
1 cup mixed frozen berries (5 ounces)
2 tablespoons 100% freshly squeezed orange juice

Place the amaranth, soy milk, ¼ teaspoon of the cinnamon, and ⅛ teaspoon of salt in a saucepan. Bring to a simmer and cook for 20 to 25 minutes, until the liquid is absorbed.

Meanwhile, place the berries, orange juice, the remaining ⅛ teaspoon cinnamon, and the remaining ⅛ teaspoon salt in a small saucepan. Cook over medium-low heat for 10 minutes. Stir occasionally, breaking up any large berries.

Divide the amaranth into 4 bowls. Top each with 2 tablespoons of the berry topping.

Nutritional Analysis

Per ¾ cup amaranth and 2 tablespoons berry topping: 239 Calories, 3 g Fat, 0.7 g Sat,

4 mg Chol, 1 g Fiber, 13 g Protein, 41 g Carb, 166 mg Sodium

Soy-Nut Pancakes with Strawberry-Banana Sauce

You can add fresh fruit to the batter and try whipped natural nut butter with a touch of honey in it as a topping.

Phase II: Maintenance
Gluten Free
Dairy Free
Quick

Serves 4
Serving Size: 3 pancakes
plus ½ cup sauce
Yield: 12 pancakes plus
2 cups sauce
Prep time: 15 minutes
Cook time: 5 to 7 minutes

1 small banana

2 cups fresh strawberries (or frozen unsweetened, thawed, with juice)

1 teaspoon honey

½ cup drained silken tofu

½ cup plain soy milk

2 tablespoons ground flaxseed

¾ cup almond flour

½ cup soy flour

2 teaspoons baking powder

Pinch kosher salt

1 teaspoon vanilla extract

1 whole omega-3 egg

Grapeseed oil for griddle

In a blender, combine the banana, strawberries, and honey. Puree for 5 to 10 seconds for a chunky sauce. Set aside sauce in a small bowl.

Without washing the blender, combine the tofu, soy milk, flaxseed, almond and soy flours, baking powder, salt, vanilla, and egg, and mix until smooth.

Preheat a griddle to 400 degrees and lightly brush with grapeseed oil. Pour approximately ¼ cup batter directly from the blender onto the griddle for each pancake. Cook pancakes until bubbles form on the surface and burst, about 4 minutes. Turn pancakes over and cook about 2 more minutes, until cooked through. Serve 3 pancakes per person with ½ cup of sauce.

Nutritional Analysis

Per 3-pancake serving: 221 Calories, 14 g Fat, 1.7 g Sat, 53 mg Chol, 5 g Fiber, 14 g Protein, 17 g Carb, 79 mg Sodium

Per ½ cup sauce: 66 Calories, 0 g Fat, 0 g Sat, 0 mg Chol, 3 g Fiber, 1 g Protein, 17 g Carb, 3 mg Sodium

Breakfast Burrito

Phase II: Maintenance
Gluten Free (with sprouted
corn or brown rice tortilla)
Dairy Free
Quick
Vegetarian

Serves 1
Serving size: 1 burrito
Prep time: 2 minutes
Cook time: 10 minutes

A quick, easy, and tasty breakfast entrée that won't leave you feeling hungry in an hour.

2 large eggs

1 tablespoon water

Pinch of freshly ground black pepper

1½ teaspoons extra-virgin olive oil

1 (8-inch) sprouted corn or brown rice tortilla

1 recipe Basic Tomato Salsa (page 167)

In a small bowl, beat the eggs with the water and pepper.

Heat the extra-virgin olive oil in a small skillet over medium heat. Add the egg mixture and stir slowly, scraping the bottom and sides of the pan. Continue cooking until the eggs reach the desired consistency.

Wrap the tortilla in foil and heat at 300 degrees F. until steaming, about 5 minutes.

Place the eggs on the warmed tortilla and top with 3 tablespoons of the salsa.

Nutritional Analysis

Per burrito: 274 Calories, 17 g Fat, 4.1 g Sat, 430 mg Chol, 2 g Fiber, 14 g Protein, 17 g Carb, 240 mg Sodium

Fruit and Nut Granola

This cereal is crunchy with nuts and seeds, and slightly sweet with honey and dried fruit. If dried blueberries are unavailable, substitute another dried fruit.

3 cups old-fashioned rolled oats

½ cup chopped raw, unsalted almonds

¼ cup chopped Brazil nuts

¼ cup raw, unsalted sunflower seeds

¼ cup flaxseed

¼ cup wheat germ

1 teaspoon ground cinnamon

Pinch of ground nutmeg

Pinch of kosher salt

3 tablespoons canned unsweetened lite coconut milk

2 tablespoons honey

1½ teaspoons vanilla extract

1 teaspoon grapeseed or other neutral-flavored oil

½ cup dried cranberries

½ cup dried blueberries

½ cup golden raisins

Phase II: Maintenance
Dairy Free
Vegetarian
Egg Free

Serves 12
Serving size: ½ cup
Yield: 6 cups
Prep time: 10 minutes
Cook time: 45 minutes

Preheat the oven to 275 degrees F.

In a large bowl, combine the oats, almonds, Brazil nuts, sunflower seeds, flaxseed, wheat germ, cinnamon, nutmeg, and salt.

In a small bowl, whisk together the coconut milk, honey, and vanilla. Drizzle over the oat and nut mixture and combine well.

Brush a sheet pan with the grapeseed oil. Transfer the granola to the sheet pan and bake for about 45 minutes, stirring every 15 minutes, until brown.

Remove from the oven and stir in the fruit. Let cool and store in an airtight container. Refrigerate after 5 days.

Nutritional Analysis

Per ½-cup serving: 219 Calories, 2.5 g Fat, 1.6 g Sat, 1 mg Chol,

7 g Fiber, 7 g Protein, 42 g Carb, 30 mg Sodium

Herbed Scrambled Egg Sandwiches on Whole-Kernel Rye Toast

Phase II: Maintenance
Gluten Free (with gluten-
free bread)
Dairy Free
Quick
Vegetarian

Serves 2
Serving size: 1 sandwich
Yield: 2 sandwiches
Prep time: 10 minutes
Cook time: 1 minute

A little different for breakfast, these sandwiches are very filling and would also make a nice light lunch. The fresh minced herbs and sun-dried tomato add variety, flavor, and color to the eggs. Be sure to use 100 percent whole kernel rye bread for a delicious gluten-free sandwich.

2 large eggs

1 tablespoon water

2 teaspoons minced sun-dried tomato (drained and patted dry if oil packed)

1 teaspoon minced chives

1 teaspoon minced parsley

1 teaspoon minced tarragon

⅛ teaspoon kosher salt

Pinch of freshly ground black pepper

1 teaspoon extra-virgin olive oil

4 (1-ounce) slices whole-kernel rye bread, toasted (see resources)

In a large bowl, whisk together the eggs, water, tomato, chives, parsley, tarragon, salt, and pepper.

Heat the extra-virgin olive oil in a small skillet over medium-high heat. Add the egg mixture and cook, stirring, until the eggs are set to the desired degree of doneness.

Lay 2 slices of the toast on a plate or cutting board. Place half the eggs on each slice. Top with the remaining 2 slices of toast. Cut each sandwich in half, and serve hot.

Nutritional Analysis

Per sandwich: 357 Calories, 9 g Fat, 1.9 g Sat, 215 mg Chol, 16 g Fiber, 12 g Protein, 54 g Carb, 832 mg Sodium

Maple Spiced Oatmeal with Currants

Steel-cut oats are the whole oat groat (the inner portion of the oat kernel) that has been cut into 2 or 3 pieces. Golden in color, they resemble mini rice particles, and their texture is firm and satisfying. This dish has a subtle maple flavor with a hint of spice. The currants add nice flavor and texture, and their size is similar to the nuggets of oats.

Phase II: Maintenance
Dairy Free
Vegetarian
Egg Free

Serves 4
Serving size: ¾ cup
Yield: 3 cups
Prep time: 5 minutes
Cook time: 30 to 35 minutes

4 cups water

1 cup steel-cut oats

½ cup currants

1 teaspoon gluten-free maple extract

½ teaspoon cinnamon

Pinch of allspice

¼ cup organic unsweetened soymilk (optional)

Bring the water to a boil in a medium saucepan. Stir in the oats. Bring to a boil, reduce the heat to low, and simmer, uncovered, for 20 minutes, stirring occasionally.

Add the currants and cook for 10 minutes. Stir frequently to prevent sticking. When the oatmeal is done, add the maple extract, cinnamon, and allspice. Add the milk if using.

Nutritional Analysis

Per ¾-cup serving: 199 Calories, 3 g Fat, 0.6 g Sat, 1 mg Chol,

5 g Fiber, 7 g Protein, 41.5 g Carb, 10 mg Sodium

Asparagus and Cheese Frittata

A classic combination of asparagus and Parmesan, with the addition of herbs and tomato.

Phase II: Maintenance
Gluten Free
Quick
Vegetarian

Serves 6
Serving size: 1 wedge
Yield: 6 wedges
Prep time: 10 minutes
Cook time: 10 minutes

½ pound asparagus, trimmed and cut into 1-inch lengths

6 large eggs

⅓ cup grated Parmesan cheese

1 tablespoon finely chopped parsley

¼ teaspoon kosher salt

¼ teaspoon freshly ground black pepper

2 tablespoons extra-virgin olive oil

¼ cup chopped tomato

1 tablespoon snipped chives

Bring a large pot of salted water to a boil. Drop in the asparagus and cook for about 2 minutes, until crisp-tender. Drain, and transfer to a bowl of ice water to stop the cooking. Drain the asparagus and set aside.

In a large bowl, beat the eggs with the cheese, parsley, salt, and pepper. Stir in the blanched asparagus.

Preheat the broiler to high.

Heat the extra-virgin olive oil in a 10-inch ovenproof skillet over medium heat. Add the egg mixture and cook, lifting the edges of the eggs as they set, allowing the uncooked egg to run underneath. Cook for 5 to 10 minutes, until the bottom is golden brown and the top is almost set, but still runny. Transfer the frittata to the broiler and cook about 1 minute, until the top is set and golden.

Remove from the oven and slide onto a plate. Garnish with the chopped tomato and chives.

Nutritional Analysis

Per wedge: 145 Calories, 11 g Fat, 3.0 g Sat, 219 mg Chol, 0 g Fiber, 9 g Protein, 2 g Carb, 260 mg Sodium

Ratatouille Omelet

This omelet is a great use for leftover Ratatouille (page 148). You can use any black olive, but Kalamata olives are recommended.

2 large eggs

1 tablespoon water

⅛ teaspoon kosher salt

Pinch of freshly ground black pepper

2 teaspoons extra-virgin olive oil

3 tablespoons Ratatouille (page 148)

2 teaspoons finely snipped chives

2 teaspoons chopped black olives (about 2 olives)

Phase II: Maintenance
Gluten Free
Dairy Free
Quick
Vegetarian

Serves 1
Serving size: 1 omelet
Yield: 1 omelet
Prep time: 5 minutes
Cook time: 5 minutes

In a large bowl, whisk together the eggs, water, salt, and pepper.

Heat the extra-virgin olive oil in a medium skillet over medium-high heat. Use a smaller pan if you prefer a thicker omelet. Add the eggs and stir until they are beginning to set on the bottom. Using a rubber spatula, lift the eggs near the edge of the pan that are set, and let most of the liquid eggs run underneath to cook.

When the eggs are nearly set, spoon the ratatouille over half of the eggs. Using a large spatula, carefully lift and then fold the other side of the omelet over the ratatouille. Turn the heat to low and continue to cook for about 1 minute, to heat the ratatouille. Slide the omelet out of the skillet onto a plate. Garnish with the snipped chives and chopped olives.

Nutritional Analysis

Per omelet: 322 Calories, 24.6 g Fat, 4.8 g Sat, 363 mg Chol,

2 g Fiber, 14 g Protein, 10 g Carb, 716 mg Sodium

Spanish Potato and Onion Tortilla

Phase II: Maintenance
Gluten Free
Dairy Free
Vegetarian

6 servings
Serving size: ⅙ tortilla
Yield: 6 slices
Prep time: 45 minutes plus
10 minutes to finish
Cook time: 20 to 25
minutes for the potatoes
and onions

This is a Spanish version of an Italian frittata, or flat omelet. The "tortilla" makes a lovely brunch or lunch entrée when cut into wedges, or for an appetizer or tapas buffet, cut into bite-size pieces. It may seem like there is a lot of olive oil in this recipe, but the potatoes do not absorb most of it.

¼ cup plus 2 tablespoons extra-virgin olive oil

2 medium onions, peeled and cut into ⅛-inch-thick slices

2 pounds Russet potatoes, peeled and cut into ⅛-inch-thick slices

1 teaspoon kosher salt

6 large eggs

½ teaspoon freshly ground black pepper

¼ teaspoon smoked Spanish paprika

Heat 2 tablespoons of the extra-virgin olive oil in a medium skillet. Add the onions and cook over medium-low heat for about 20 minutes, until soft and starting to turn golden brown.

Heat the remaining ¼ cup extra-virgin olive oil in a 10-inch skillet, preferably nonstick. Add the potatoes, in batches, in a single layer. Cook for about 2 minutes, turning once, until the potatoes turn light brown and are crisp on the edges. When done, remove each batch to paper towels to drain. Sprinkle the potatoes with ½ teaspoon of the salt. Pour all but 1 tablespoon of the olive oil out of the skillet and set the skillet aside for cooking the eggs.

After the potatoes and onions are precooked, preheat the broiler to high.

In a medium bowl, lightly beat the eggs with the remaining ½ teaspoon salt, the pepper, and paprika. Add the cooked potatoes and onions.

Heat the reserved oil in the skillet used for the potatoes over medium-high heat. When the oil is hot, add the beaten eggs. Shake the pan to distribute the eggs.

Cook for about 1 minute, lifting the cooked edges of the eggs to allow the liquid egg to run underneath. Turn the heat to low and cook the tortilla for about 5 minutes, until brown on the bottom.

When the eggs look almost fully set, place the skillet under the broiler. Cook for about 3 to 5 minutes, until all the egg is cooked and the tortilla is a deep golden brown.

Slice into 6 wedges, and serve hot or at room temperature.

Nutritional Analysis

Per ⅙ tortilla: 256 Calories, 11 g Fat, 2.3 g Sat, 180 mg Chol,

3.6 g Fiber, 10 g Protein, 25 g Carb, 396 mg Sodium

Sweet Potato Hash with Eggs

A nice variation on corned beef hash, this combination of sweet potatoes and peppers is seasoned with a pinch of paprika. It makes a delicious weekend breakfast or vegetarian supper.

Phase II: Maintenance
Gluten Free
Dairy Free

Serves 4
Serving size: ½ cup hash plus 1 egg
Yield: 2 cups hash plus 4 eggs
Prep time: 20 minutes
Cook time: 25 minutes

2 medium (about 1 pound) sweet potatoes, peeled and finely diced

¼ cup plus 1 teaspoon extra-virgin olive oil

¾ cup finely diced red bell pepper (about 1 medium pepper)

¾ cup finely diced green bell pepper (about 1 medium pepper)

½ cup finely diced red onion (about 1 small onion)

2 teaspoons minced garlic

1 teaspoon minced jalapeño pepper

½ teaspoon kosher salt

1 teaspoon minced oregano

½ teaspoon freshly ground black pepper

Pinch of paprika

4 large eggs

Bring a large pot of salted water to a boil. Cook the sweet potatoes for about 3 minutes, until crisp-tender. Drain and set aside.

Heat ½ cup of the extra-virgin olive oil in a large skillet over medium heat. Add the red and green pepper, onion, garlic, jalapeño pepper, and salt. Cook for about 10 minutes, stirring frequently, until the vegetables are soft. Increase the heat to medium-high and add the cooked sweet potatoes, oregano, black pepper, and paprika. Cook for about 10 minutes, stirring frequently, until the vegetables are soft and lightly brown.

Meanwhile, heat the remaining 1 teaspoon extra-virgin olive oil in a large, preferably nonstick, skillet over medium heat. One at a time, break the eggs into a small bowl, then slide them into the skillet. Cook until the whites are set. Gently turn the eggs over and cook for about 1 minute for over easy, or about 2 minutes for over well.

Nutritional Analysis

Per ½ cup hash plus 1 egg: 294 Calories, 20 g Fat, 3.7 g Sat,

215 mg Chol, 4 g Fiber, 8 g Protein, 21 g Carb, 332 mg Sodium

Vegetable Omelet with Manchego Cheese

Phase II: Maintenance
Gluten Free
Quick
Vegetarian

Serves 1
Serving size: 1 omelet
Prep time: 10 minutes
Cook time: 5 minutes

A satisfying entrée served at breakfast, lunch, or brunch. The Manchego cheese adds a smooth, rich flavor to the omelet.

3 teaspoons extra-virgin olive oil

1 tablespoon diced green bell pepper

1 tablespoon diced red onion

2 large eggs

1 tablespoon water

¼ teaspoon kosher salt

Pinch of freshly ground black pepper

The UltraMetabolism Cookbook

2 tablespoons grated Manchego cheese (½ ounce)

2 tablespoons chopped tomato

1 medium scallion, chopped (2 teaspoons), for garnish

Heat 1 teaspoon of the extra-virgin olive oil in a small skillet. Add the green pepper and onion and cook for about 3 to 4 minutes, until tender. When cooked, remove from the pan and set the skillet aside for cooking the eggs.

Meanwhile, in a medium bowl, beat together the eggs, water, salt, and pepper.

Heat the remaining 2 teaspoons of extra-virgin olive oil in the small skillet over medium heat. Add the eggs and stir until they begin to set on the bottom and around the edges. Using a spatula, lift the edge of the eggs that are set and let the liquid eggs run underneath to cook.

When the eggs are nearly set throughout, spread the green pepper, onion, grated cheese, and tomato over half of the egg circle. Using a large spatula, carefully lift and fold the other side of the omelet over the vegetables and cheese. Turn the heat to low and continue to cook for about 1 minute, to melt the cheese and heat the vegetables. Slide the omelet out of the skillet onto a plate.

Garnish with the scallions.

Nutritional Analysis

Per omelet: 347 Calories, 27 g Fat, 7.0 g Sat, 376 mg Chol, 1 g Fiber, 17 g Protein, 6 g Carb, 672 mg Sodium

Apple Sauce

Phase II: Maintenance
Gluten Free
Dairy Free
Vegetarian
Egg Free

Serves 4
Serving size: ½ cup
Yield: 2 cups
Prep time: 15 minutes
Cook time: 40 minutes

For a more complex apple flavor, use a mix of apples, such as Granny Smith, Gala, and Fuji, in this slightly sweet sauce with the warming flavors of cinnamon and allspice.

4 large apples (about 2 pounds), peeled, cored, and cut into chunks
1 cup water
½ teaspoon cinnamon
Small pinch of allspice
½ teaspoon fresh lemon juice

Place the apples in a large pan with the water. Cover and bring to a boil over medium-high heat. Reduce heat to medium and cook the apples until they are soft, about 20 to 25 minutes.

When the apples are cooked, remove only the apples to the bowl of a food processor, fitted with a metal blade, leaving any cooking liquid in the pan.

Bring the remaining liquid in the pan to a boil over high heat until it reduces to about 1 or 2 tablespoons.

Add the reduced liquid from the pan to the food processor along with the cinnamon, allspice, and lemon juice, and process to the desired consistency.

Nutritional Analysis

Per ½-cup serving: 110 Calories, 0 g Fat, 0 g Sat, 0 mg Chol, 5 g Fiber, 1 g Protein, 29 g Carb, 2 mg Sodium

Basil Vinaigrette

Pair with any plain grilled chicken breast or fillet of fish. In the heat of summer, drizzle over a platter of garden-fresh ripe red tomatoes.

3 cups basil leaves, moderately packed

¾ cup extra-virgin olive oil

3 tablespoons red wine vinegar

2 medium cloves garlic, chopped

½ teaspoon kosher salt

½ teaspoon freshly ground black pepper

Phase II

Phase II: Maintenance
Gluten Free
Dairy Free
Quick
Vegetarian
Egg Free

Serves 8
Serving size: 2 tablespoons
Yield: 1 cup
Prep time: 10 minutes
Cook time: none

Combine all ingredients in the bowl of a food processor fitted with a metal blade. Process until smooth, scraping the sides of the bowl as necessary.

Nutritional Analysis
Per 2-tablespoon serving: 196 Calories, 21 g Fat, 3.0 g Sat, 0 mg Chol,

1 g Fiber, 1 g Protein, 1 g Carb, 121 mg Sodium

Lemon-Mustard Vinaigrette

Use this tangy, slightly sweet, versatile vinaigrette on everything from dark, strongly flavored greens to pork chops fresh off the grill.

2 tablespoons fresh lemon juice

1½ teaspoons honey

1 teaspoon Dijon mustard

1 teaspoon minced garlic (1 medium clove)

½ teaspoon kosher salt

¼ teaspoon freshly ground black pepper

½ cup extra-virgin olive oil

Phase II: Maintenance
Gluten Free
Dairy Free
Quick
Vegetarian
Egg Free

Serves 5
Serving size: 2 tablespoons
Yield: about ⅔ cup
Prep time: 10 minutes
Cook time: none

In a small bowl, combine all ingredients except the extra-virgin olive oil. Slowly whisk in the extra-virgin olive oil until the dressing is slightly thickened. Alternatively, place all ingredients in a jar with a tight-fitting lid and shake until well combined.

Nutritional Analysis

Per 2-tablespoon serving: 204 Calories, 22 g Fat, 3.2 g Sat, 0 mg Chol,

0 g Fiber, 0 g Protein, 3 g Carb, 217 mg Sodium

Raspberry Vinaigrette

The tart raspberry vinaigrette is tasty drizzled on a green salad or grilled poultry.

Phase II: Maintenance
Gluten Free
Dairy Free
Quick
Vegetarian
Egg Free

Serves 5
Serving size: 2 tablespoons
Yield: about ⅔ cup
Prep time: 5 minutes
Cook time: none

2 tablespoons raspberry vinegar

1 teaspoon whole-grain mustard

½ teaspoon minced garlic

½ teaspoon kosher salt

¼ teaspoon freshly ground black pepper

½ cup extra-virgin olive oil

In a medium bowl, whisk together the vinegar, mustard, garlic, salt, and pepper. Slowly whisk in the extra-virgin olive oil until slightly thickened. Alternatively, place all ingredients in a jar with a tight-fitting lid and shake until well combined.

Nutritional Analysis

Per 2-tablespoon serving: 204 Calories, 22 g Fat, 3.1 g Sat, 0 mg Chol,

0 g Fiber, 0 g Protein, 0 g Carb, 216 mg Sodium

Sherry-Walnut Vinaigrette

This vinaigrette is prepared with a delicious combination of olive and walnut oils, tangy lemon juice, and sherry vinegar.

2 tablespoons sherry wine vinegar

2 teaspoons fresh lemon juice

¾ teaspoon kosher salt

¼ teaspoon freshly ground black pepper

6 tablespoons walnut oil

2 tablespoons extra-virgin olive oil

Phase II: Maintenance
Gluten Free
Dairy Free
Quick
Vegetarian
Egg Free

Serves 5
Serving size: 2 tablespoons
Yield: about ⅔ cup
Prep time: 5 minutes
Cook time: none

In a medium bowl, mix together the vinegar, lemon juice, salt, and pepper. Slowly whisk in the walnut and extra-virgin olive oils until slightly thickened. Alternatively, place all ingredients in a jar with a tight-fitting lid and shake until well combined.

Nutritional Analysis

Per 2-tablespoon serving: 195 Calories, 22 g Fat, 2.3 g Sat, 0 mg Chol,

0 g Fiber, 0 g Protein, 0 g Carb, 288 mg Sodium

Sherry-White Wine Vinaigrette

The sherry vinegar adds a nice background flavor, and it is especially good on a mixed green salad.

1 small clove garlic, minced

½ teaspoon kosher salt

¼ teaspoon freshly ground black pepper

1 tablespoon sherry wine vinegar

1 tablespoon white wine vinegar

½ teaspoon Dijon mustard

Phase II: Maintenance
Gluten Free
Dairy Free
Quick
Vegetarian
Egg Free

Serves 5
Serving size: 2 tablespoons
Yield: about ⅔ cup
Prep time: 10 minutes
Cook time: none

½ teaspoon fresh lemon juice

½ cup extra-virgin olive oil

In a medium bowl, whisk together the garlic, salt, pepper, vinegars, mustard, and lemon juice. Slowly whisk in the extra-virgin olive oil until slightly thickened. Alternatively, place all ingredients in a jar with a tight-fitting lid and shake until well combined.

Nutritional Analysis

Per 2-tablespoon serving: 203 Calories, 22 g Fat, 3.2 g Sat, 0 mg Chol,

0 g Fiber, 0 g Protein, 0 g Carb, 199 mg Sodium

Cilantro Buttermilk Dressing

Phase II: Maintenance
Gluten Free
Quick
Vegetarian
Egg Free

Serves 4
Serving size: 2 tablespoons
Yield: about ½ cup
Prep time: 10 minutes
Cook time: none

Slightly spicy, with a Southwestern touch, this sauce is perfect atop Chicken Cutlets with Cornmeal Crust (page 214), as a salad dressing, or as a dip with fresh, raw vegetables or corn chips.

½ cup nonfat cultured buttermilk

2 tablespoons reduced-fat sour cream

2 teaspoons minced cilantro

2 teaspoons minced chives

2 teaspoons fresh lime juice

1 teaspoon minced jalapeño pepper

1 medium clove garlic, minced

In a medium bowl, whisk all ingredients together. Refrigerate until ready to serve.

Nutritional Analysis

Per 2-tablespoon serving: 17 Calories, 0 g Fat, 0.6 g Sat, 4 mg Chol,

0 g Fiber, 2 g Protein, 3 g Carb, 39 mg Sodium

Cilantro-Mint Dipping Sauce

Herbaceous, spicy, and slightly sweet, this sauce has a beautiful, bright green color. If you prefer less heat, reduce the amount of jalapeño pepper. Serve with roasted shrimp, grilled fish, or chicken.

1½ cups lightly packed cilantro leaves and some tender stems

1 cup lightly packed mint leaves

¼ cup plus 2 tablespoons fresh lime juice

1 tablespoon honey

4 teaspoons minced jalapeño pepper

2 teaspoons minced ginger

1 teaspoon minced garlic

Pinch of kosher salt

Combine all the ingredients in the bowl of a food processor fitted with a metal blade. Process until smooth, occasionally stopping to scrape down the bowl.

Nutritional Analysis

Per 2-tablespoon serving: 11 Calories, 0 g Fat, 0 g Sat, 0 mg Chol,

0 g Fiber, 0 g Protein, 2.5 g Carb, 23 mg Sodium

Phase II: Maintenance
Gluten Free
Dairy Free
Quick
Vegetarian
Egg Free

Serves 6
Serving size: 2 tablespoons
Yield: ¾ cup
Prep time: 15 minutes
Cook time: none

Citrus Vinaigrette

Phase II: Maintenance
Gluten Free
Dairy Free
Quick
Vegetarian
Egg Free

Serves 5
Serving size: 2 tablespoons
Yield: about ⅔ cup
Prep time: 10 minutes
Cook time: none

This subtly flavored vinaigrette contains orange, with a hint of lemon. Serve on Roasted Beet Salad with Warm Goat Cheese (page 196) or a mixed green salad.

½ teaspoon orange zest

2 tablespoons fresh orange juice

2 tablespoons fresh lemon juice

1 teaspoon Dijon mustard

½ teaspoon kosher salt

½ teaspoon freshly ground black pepper

½ cup extra-virgin olive oil

In a small bowl, mix the orange zest, orange juice, lemon juice, mustard, salt, and pepper. Slowly whisk in the extra-virgin olive oil until the dressing is slightly thickened. Alternatively, place all ingredients in a jar with a tight-fitting lid and shake until well combined.

Nutritional Analysis

Per 2-tablespoon serving: 207 Calories, 22 g Fat, 3.1 g Sat, 0 mg Chol,

0 g Fiber, 0 g Protein, 1 g Carb, 205 mg Sodium

Creamy White Wine Vinaigrette

A change from typical vinaigrettes, this version is a creamy dressing made without cream.

3 tablespoons white wine vinegar

1 tablespoon Homemade Mayonnaise (page 258) or organic soy mayonnaise

1 teaspoon minced garlic (about 1 medium clove)

½ teaspoon Dijon mustard

½ teaspoon kosher salt

½ teaspoon freshly ground black pepper

½ cup extra-virgin olive oil

Phase II: Maintenance
Gluten Free
Dairy Free
Quick
Vegetarian
Egg Free (with soy mayonnaise)

Serves 6
Serving size: 2 tablespoons
Yield: ¾ cup
Prep time: 5 minutes
Cook time: none

In a small bowl, mix the vinegar, mayonnaise, garlic, mustard, salt, and pepper. Slowly whisk in the extra-virgin olive oil until the dressing is slightly thickened. Alternatively, place all ingredients in a jar with a tight-fitting lid and shake until well combined.

Nutritional Analysis

Per 2-tablespoon serving: 185 Calories, 21 g Fat, 3.0 g Sat, 2 mg Chol,

0 g Fiber, 0 g Protein, 0 g Carb, 176 mg Sodium

Garlicky Cucumber-Yogurt Sauce

Use as a dip with fresh vegetables or pita bread toasts.

Phase II: Maintenance
Dairy Free (with soy yogurt)
Gluten Free
Vegetarian
Egg Free

Serves 8
Serving size: ¼ cup
Yield: 2 cups
Prep time: 1¼ hours
Cook time: none

1¼ cups nonfat plain yogurt or plain soy yogurt

1 tablespoon extra-virgin olive oil

1 tablespoon finely chopped mint

1 tablespoon minced scallion (1 small scallion)

2 teaspoons minced garlic

½ teaspoon kosher salt

1 cup finely chopped seeded cucumber, drained of excess liquid

Drain the yogurt by lining a strainer or colander with a double layer of paper towels. Spoon the yogurt into the paper towel–lined strainer and place the strainer over a bowl. Refrigerate for at least 1 hour to allow the liquid to drain from the yogurt into the bowl.

When the yogurt has drained, discard the liquid and place the yogurt in a medium bowl. Add the extra-virgin olive oil, mint, scallion, garlic, and salt and stir well to combine. Add the cucumber to the sauce just before serving.

Nutritional Analysis

Per ¼-cup serving: 35 Calories, 2 g Fat, 0.3 g Sat, 1 mg Chol, 0 g Fiber, 2 g Protein, 4 g Carb, 142 mg Sodium

Hazelnut Vinaigrette

Steep the hazelnuts in the dressing for maximum flavor. Excellent on many greens, this vinaigrette is truly wonderful on Baby Arugula, Shaved Fennel, and Cranberry Salad (page 192).

Phase II: Maintenance
Gluten Free
Dairy Free
Quick
Vegetarian
Egg Free

Serves 6
Serving size: 2 tablespoons
Yield: about ¾ cup
Prep time: 15 minutes
Cook time: none

6 tablespoons coarsely chopped hazelnuts

2 tablespoons fresh lemon juice

1 teaspoon minced shallot

½ teaspoon minced garlic

½ teaspoon Dijon mustard

½ teaspoon kosher salt

½ teaspoon freshly ground black pepper

¼ cup hazelnut oil

¼ cup extra-virgin olive oil

Toast the hazelnuts in a small skillet over medium heat for about 3 to 4 minutes. Stir frequently and watch closely to prevent burning. When toasted, remove the nuts to a plate to cool.

In a medium bowl, combine the lemon juice, shallot, garlic, mustard, salt, and pepper. Slowly whisk in the oils until the dressing is slightly thickened. Add the toasted hazelnuts. Alternatively, place all ingredients in a jar with a tight-fitting lid and shake until well combined. Let the dressing rest for 30 minutes to allow the hazelnuts to absorb the flavor.

Nutritional Analysis

Per 2-tablespoon serving: 129 Calories, 13 g Fat, 1.0 g Sat, 0 mg Chol,

1 g Fiber, 1 g Protein, 2 g Carb, 166 mg Sodium

Homemade Mayonnaise

Phase II: Maintenance
Gluten Free
Dairy Free
Quick
Vegetarian

Serves 8
Serving size: 2 tablespoons
Yield: 1 cup
Prep time: 5 minutes
Cook time: none

Elegant, delicious, and flavorful, this homemade mayonnaise takes a little more time but is well worth the effort.

1 large egg
1 tablespoon fresh lemon juice
½ teaspoon kosher salt
Pinch of ground red pepper
¾ cup extra-virgin olive oil

Combine the egg, lemon juice, salt, and pepper in the bowl of a food processor. With the machine running, add the extra-virgin olive oil in a slow stream until the mixture is thick and light colored.

Nutritional Analysis

Per 2-tablespoon serving: 95 Calories, 11 g Fat, 1.6 g Sat, 0 mg Chol,

0 g Fiber, 0 g Protein, 0 g Carb, 64 mg Sodium

The UltraMetabolism Cookbook

Miso Dressing

This dressing is delicious spooned over Citrus-Marinated Cod (page 205), adding some tang and heat, and is also quite good on a mixed green salad.

2 tablespoons rice wine vinegar

1 tablespoon light gluten-free miso paste

½ tablespoon low-sodium wheat-free tamari

1 teaspoon dark sesame oil

¾ teaspoon grated fresh ginger

¼ teaspoon Thai Kitchen Red Chili Paste

¼ cup light sesame oil

Phase II: Maintenance
Gluten Free
Dairy Free
Quick
Vegetarian
Egg Free

Serves 4
Serving size: 2 tablespoons
Yield: ½ cup
Prep time: 10 minutes
Cook time: none

In a medium bowl, whisk together the vinegar, miso paste, tamari, dark sesame oil, ginger, garlic, and red chili paste. Use the back of a spoon if necessary to mash and dissolve the miso paste. Slowly whisk in the light sesame oil until the dressing is slightly thickened.

Nutritional Analysis

Per 2-tablespoon serving: 142 Calories, 15 g Fat, 2.2 g Sat, 0 mg Chol,

0 g Fiber, 1 g Protein, 1.6 g Carb, 200 mg Sodium

Orange-White Wine Vinaigrette

Phase II: Maintenance
Gluten Free
Dairy Free
Quick
Vegetarian
Egg Free

Serves 6
Serving size: 2 tablespoons
Yield: generous ¾ cup
Prep time: 15 minutes
Cook time: none

With a pleasant, sweet citrus flavor, this vinaigrette is especially good on a grilled chicken breast or a piece of firm white-fleshed fish.

½ cup 100% freshly squeezed orange juice

2 tablespoons white wine vinegar

2 small cloves garlic, minced

1 teaspoon Dijon mustard

½ teaspoon kosher salt

½ teaspoon freshly ground black pepper

6 tablespoons extra-virgin olive oil

Place the orange juice in a small pan and bring to a boil. Continue to boil until reduced in volume by half. Set aside to cool.

In a small bowl, combine the reduced orange juice, vinegar, garlic, mustard, salt, and pepper. Slowly whisk in the extra-virgin olive oil until the dressing is slightly thickened. Alternatively, place all ingredients in a jar with a tight-fitting lid and shake until well combined.

Nutritional Analysis

Per 2-tablespoon serving: 137 Calories, 14 g Fat, 2 g Sat, 0 mg Chol,

0 g Fiber, 0 g Protein, 2.3 g Carb, 180 mg Sodium

The UltraMetabolism Cookbook

Sicilian-Style Sweet and Sour Sauce

Tomato-based, with the briny taste of olives and capers, this Sicilian-inspired sauce has a hint of natural sweetness from the raisins and balsamic vinegar. Served this with grilled fish or chicken.

Phase II: Maintenance
Gluten Free
Dairy Free
Quick
Vegetarian
Egg Free

Serves 4
Serving size: ¼ cup
Yield: 1 cup
Prep time: 15 minutes
Cook time: 20 minutes

2 tablespoons extra-virgin olive oil

¼ cup finely chopped red onion

¼ cup finely chopped celery

1 medium clove garlic, minced

1 cup drained canned whole tomatoes, finely chopped

2 tablespoons raisins

2 tablespoons chopped brine-cured green olives

1 tablespoon chopped brine-cured black olives

1 tablespoon capers

¼ teaspoon kosher salt

¼ teaspoon freshly ground black pepper

1 tablespoon pine nuts

1 tablespoon chopped parsley

1 teaspoon balsamic vinegar

1 tablespoon thinly sliced basil

Heat the extra-virgin olive oil in a small saucepan over medium heat. Add the onion and celery and cook for about 5 minutes, until softened. Add the garlic and cook for 30 seconds. Stir in the tomatoes (discarding any juice that has accumulated) along with the raisins, olives, capers, salt, and pepper. After 5 minutes add the pine nuts, parsley, and balsamic vinegar. Cook an additional 3 to 5 minutes, until the sauce is thick. Stir in the basil and serve.

Nutritional Analysis

Per ¼-cup serving: 189 Calories, 16 g Fat, 2.2 g Sat, 0 mg Chol,

1 g Fiber, 1 g Protein, 10 g Carb, 372 mg Sodium

Across the grain (as in "cut across the grain of the meat"): Refers to cutting meat perpendicular to the meat fibers. Cutting this way increases tenderness. You can easily tell the "grain" of the meat by looking at it.

Additives: Chemical compounds added to foods usually for the purpose of preservation or altering the flavor or color of the ingredients. These are not part of a whole-foods diet and should be avoided as much as possible.

Bake: A technique of cooking in an oven by applying dry heat evenly throughout.

Bisque: A thick creamy soup. It often, but not always, contains seafood.

Blanch/blanched (as in "blanched almonds" or "blanch the vegetables"): A process in which food is briefly plunged into boiling water for a moment then immediately transferred to ice water to stop the cooking process.

Braise: Preparing food by browning then cooking slowly in a small amount of liquid in a covered pan either in an oven or on a stovetop.

Brine-cured (as in "brine-cured olives"): Soaked or preserved in brine, a water mixture saturated with salt.

Brown (as in "pan-browned" or "brown the top of the meat"): Briefly frying meat until the surface becomes brown. This enhances flavor both by bringing it out on the surface of the meat and trapping juice inside the meat.

Caramelized: Cooking so that natural sugar in the food is brought out.

Cold-pressed/expeller-pressed oils: Processes for obtaining oils from seeds or nuts in a way that is free from chemical agents. This keeps them cleaner and helps retain vital phytonutrients.

Dairy free: Made without dairy products of any kind.

Egg free: Made without eggs.

Fold (as in "gently fold the liquid ingredients into the dry products"): Gently turning over ingredients with a spatula instead of vigorously stirring them.

Free-range: The term applied to feed animals (such as cows, chickens, or pigs) that were not raised exclusively in a stockyard or feedlot, but rather allowed to roam free on the range or in the pasture.

Gluten free: Made without gluten, which is found in common grains such as wheat, barley, rye, spelt, kamut, and oats.

Glycemic load (GL): A measure of how quickly sugar from foods enters your bloodstream. Low-glycemic-load foods are much more healthful than high-glycemic-load foods.

Grass-fed: The term applied to feed animals (such as cows, chickens, or pigs) that have been raised, at least partially, in the pasture. These animals are usually given less antibiotics and their meat tends to be leaner, hence they are healthier to eat.

Grass-finished: The term applied to feed animals (such as cows, chicken, or pigs) that have been raised exclusively in pasture. Usually these animals aren't given any antibiotics and their meat is leanest of all. These are the healthiest animals to eat.

High-fructose corn syrup: A highly processed form of sugar that permeates your cell walls without any work from the body. Its use in food is directly correlated with the rise in obesity. It is to be avoided at all costs.

Hydrogenated oils: Man-made fat substitutes that are poisonous to human biology. They are to be avoided at all costs.

IgE allergy: An immediate and severe food allergy that causes an anaphylactic reaction.

IgG allergy: A delayed and less severe food allergy that is caused by a "leaky gut." IgG allergies manifest themselves as any number of health or mood problems.

Julienne: Cutting food into thin sticks with a knife or mandolin.

Leaky gut (altered intestinal permeability): A condition caused by eating foods to which you are sensitive that results in partially digested food particles "leaking" through your intestinal lining and setting off IgG allergies (see above).

Monounsaturated fats: The type of fat found in olive oil, walnut oil, and grapeseed oil. These are healthful oils to consume.

Nutrigenomics: The science of how nutrition turns on and off certain genes—of how food contains information, not just calories.

Omega-3 fats: Part of the polyunsaturated

fat family, these are the most healthful of all fats. Unfortunately, they are also fats in which American diets are notoriously low. Include many omega-3 fats in your diet.

Organic/certified organic: Organic foods have been raised in close harmony with the local ecology in which they are grown. This includes a limit on the amount and types of pesticides used. Certified organic products are held to strict standards by the National Organics Standards Board. These standards include strict rules regarding what pesticides can be used.

Quick: Recipes that take less than 30 minutes to prepare and cook.

Parchment paper (for baking): Special paper that doesn't burn or contaminate food when it is cooked in the oven.

Phytonutrient index: A measure of the amount of phytonutrients in a given food.

Phytonutrients: Chemicals in plant food that are very healthful for the human body. This is the "medicine" in your food.

Polyunsaturated fats: Highly unsaturated fats usually of plant origin. Some of these, like sesame oil, are healthful in limited amounts.

Pulse (as in "pulse in a food processor"): Repeatedly turning on and off food processor or blender to mix food.

Purée: Blending food until it is a fine substance. Often done with soups.

Preservatives: Chemical additives put in processed foods for the specific purpose of prolonging shelf life (i.e. "preserving" them). These are not a part of a wholefoods diet and should be avoided as much as possible.

Reduction (as in "to reduce a sauce" or "the apricot nectar reduction"): Cooking water or other liquid out of a sauce to enhance concentration and flavor.

Refined grain: A grain that has been processed so that the bran and germ (two of the most healthful parts of the grain) have been removed so that only the starch (or sugar) is left. Flour and sugar products are refined grains. Generally they should be avoided.

Rest (as in "let the meat rest"): Letting meat sit after it is cooked. This helps keep juice in the meat.

Roast: A method of cooking with dry heat in an oven.

Saturated fats: These fats, found mainly in animal products, break down into two basic categories: good saturated fats and bad saturated fats. Good saturated fats include coconut oil.

Sauté: To cook food quickly in a small amount of fat or oil, until brown, in a skillet or sauté pan over direct heat.

Sear (as in "pan-seared" or "sear the meat"): To brown meat quickly over high heat usually under a broiler, on a grill, or over a stovetop.

Sprouted grain: A grain that has been soaked in water or has otherwise sprouted so that the plant is starting to grow from it. These can be healthful, but should be eaten in limited amounts.

Toasted (as in "toasted nuts"): Lightly cooked. Helps bring out flavor.

Trans fats: Another term for hydrogenated oil (see above).

Whole grain: The most healthful form of grain. This is the fruit of plants (such as oats, wheat, and quinoa) that were once wild. Whole grains contain the bran, germ, and endosperm. Include many whole grains in your diet.

Whisk: Rapidly beat together ingredients using a wire whisk or some similar tool.

Tools for Healthy Living and Relaxation

Yoga and Relaxation Tools

There are many wonderful resources available to help you activate the relaxation response and reduce stress. Below is a selection of some of the best sources of CDs, lifestyle products (such as biofeedback tools), and saunas.

Health Journeys

www.healthjourneys.com
Resources for self-healing, including guided imagery tapes

Natural Journeys

www.naturaljourneys.com
Healthy lifestyle DVDs and videos including Pilates, yoga, tai chi, fitness, meditation, and self-healing

The Relaxation Company

www.therelaxationcompany.com
Music and relaxation CDs

Padma Media: Products That Support an Awakened Life

www.padmamedia.com

Home Biofeedback Tools

Wild Divine

www.wilddivine.com
Their computer guided relaxation software, Healing Rhythms, is a 15 step biofeedback program to learn the tools to help build a happy mind and healthy body.

Resperate

www.resperate.com
A personal, small biofeedback device to train yourself to relax

Stress Eraser

www.stresseraser.com
A home monitor of heart rate variability that can train you to activate the relaxation response

Emwave

www.emwave.com
A personal stress reliever also using heart rate variability to balance your nervous system from the developers of Heart Math

Saunas for Detoxification

Sunlight Saunas
www.sunlightsaunas.com
My preferred source of far-infrared saunas

High Tech Health
www.hightechhealth.com
Another source of far-infrared saunas

Home Testing

Direct Laboratory Services, Inc.
www.directabs.com

Home Allergy Testing
www.yorktest.com

Home Hair Analysis
www.bodybalance.com

Food Resources

Organic Essentials
You'll find a vast array of organic food products, home care, healthcare, kitchenware, pet care. and other valuable resources from these sites:

The Organic Food Pages
www.theorganicpages.com

Shop by Organic
www.shopbyorganics.com

Oraganics
www.oraganic.com

EfoodPantry.com
www.efoodpantry.com

Organic Provisions
www.orgfood.com

Organic Planet
www.organic-planet.com

Sun Organic Farm
www.sunorganicfarm.com

Shop Natural
www.shopnatural.com

Green for Good
www.greenforgood.com

Produce

Diamond Organics
www.diamondorganics.com
Mail-order, high-quality organic produce and raw foods

Earthbound Farms
www.earthboundfarm.com
Fresh, packaged organic produce

Small Planet Foods
www.cfarm.com
Home site of Cascadian Farms and Muir Glen—organic frozen and canned vegetables and fruits

Maine Coast Sea Vegetables
www.seaveg.com
Variety of sea vegetables, including some organically certified types

Organic Frozen Foods

Cascadian Farms
www.cfarm.com
Great source of organic frozen fruit and vegetables for those in a hurry

Stahlbush Island Farms, Inc.
www.stahlbush.com

Organic Vegetable Broth

Pacific Foods
www.pacificfoods.com

Imagine Foods
www.imaginefoods.com

Meat, Poultry, Eggs, and Dairy

Eat Wild
www.eatwild.com
Information and ordering site for grass-fed meat and dairy products

Organic Valley
www.organicvalley.com
Organic meats, dairy, eggs, and produce from 600-plus member-owned organic farms

Peaceful Pastures
www.peacefulpastures.com
Grass-fed and grass-finished meat, poultry, and dairy products

Raised Right Poultry
www.raisedright.com
Certified organic, free-range poultry

Applegate Farms
www.applegatefarms.com
Packaged organic poultry, meats, and deli products

Pete and Gerry's Organic Eggs
www.peterandgerrys.com
Organic omega-3 eggs

Stonyfield Farm
www.stonyfield.com
Certified organic dairy products and soy yogurt

Horizon Organic
www.horizonorganic.com
Variety of certified organic dairy products, including cheeses

Fish

Vital Choice Seafood
www.vitalchoice.com
Selection of fresh, frozen, and canned wild salmon

Ecofish, Inc.
www.ecofish.com
Environmentally responsible seafood products and information

Crown Prince Natural
www.crownprince.com
Wild-caught, sustainably harvested specialty canned seafood

Sea Bear
www.seabear.com
Wild salmon jerky for a convenient snack

Nuts, Seeds and Oils

Barlean's Organic Oils
www.barleans.com
Organic oils and ground flaxseed

Omega Nutrition
www.omeganutrition.com
Variety of organic oils, flax, and hempseed
products

Spectrum Naturals
www.spectrumorganic.com
Extensive line of high-quality oils, vinegars,
flax products, and culinary resources

Maranatha
www.nspiredfoods.com
Organic nut and seed butters

Once Again Nut Butter
www.onceagainnutbutter.com
Organic nut and seed butters

Beans and Legumes

Eden Foods
www.edenfoods.com
Complete line of organic dried and canned
beans

Westbrae Natural
www.westbrae.com
Full variety of organic beans and vegetarian
products (soups, condiments, pastas, etc.)

ShariAnn's Organics
www.shariannsorganic.com
Organic beans, refried beans, soups, and
more

Grains

Arrowhead Mills
www.arrowheadmills.com
Organic grains including many gluten-free
choices

Lundberg Family Farms
www.lundberg.com
Organic grains and gluten free items such as
wild rice

Hodgson Mill, Inc.
www.hodgsonmill.com
Complete line of whole grains including
many gluten-free grains

Mestemacher Breads
They offer a whole-kernel rye bread as well
as a few other whole-grain breads. They
don't have a Web site, but you can look
them up online and find many retailers
who sell their products.

Shiloh Farms
www.shilohfarms.net
Organic whole grains, sprouted grains, and
gluten-free items

Spices, Seasonings, Sauces, Soups, and Such

Spice Hunter
www.spicehunter.com
Complete line of organic spices

Frontier Herbs
www.frontiernaturalbrands.com
Extensive line of organic spices, seasonings,
baking flavors and extracts, dried foods, teas,
and culinary gadgets

Rapunzel Pure Organics
www.rapunzel.com
Great selection of seasonings, such as Herb-amare made with sea salt and organic herbs

Seeds of Change
www.seedsofchange.com
Organic tomato sauces, salsas, and more

Edward and Sons Trading Co.
www.edwardandsons.com
Extensive line of vegetarian organic food products including miso, sauces, brown rice crackers, etc.

Pacific Natural Foods
www.pacificfoods.com
Organic and gluten-free broths, soups, ready-to-eat meals, and beverages

Imagine Foods
www.imaginefoods.com
Certified organic gluten-free stocks and soups

Flavorganics
www.flavorganics.com
Full product line of certified organic pure flavor extracts

Beverages

Nondairy, Gluten-Free Beverages

Westbrae Westsoy (unsweetened soy milk)
www.westbrae.com

Imagine Foods (Soy Dream)
www.imaginefoods.com

White Wave (Silk soy beverage)
www.whitewave.com

Pacific Natural Foods (Select soy almond, hazelnut, and rice beverages)
www.pacificfoods.com

Whole Soy Co. (unsweetened soy yogurt)
www.wholesoyco.com

Organic Herbal Teas

Mighty Leaf Teas
www.mightyleaf.com

Choice Organic Teas
www.choiceorganicteas.com

Yogi Teas
www.yogitea.com

Republic of Tea
www.republicoftea.com

Numi Tea
www.numitea.com

Nutritionally Oriented Doctors and Organizations

The Institute for Functional Medicine
www.functionalmedicine.org

The American Academy of Environmental Medicine
www.aaem.com

The American College for Advancement in Medicine
www.acam.org

Web Sites
For a full listing of helpful health Web sites and resources, see www.ultrawellness.com

Download The UltraMetabolism Cookbook
Companion Guide to Boost Your Success

I've put together a guide that you can download at no charge that includes several items that I didn't have enough room for in the book. To get the most out of the program, I suggest you download this guide before starting the program. The guide includes:

- **Helpful Trackers**—A handy set of charts so you can track how much your health and weight improves as you reduce your toxicity and inflammation during the program;

- **Handy Checklists**—A series of checklists that will allow you to easily keep track of all the steps you should taking during the preparation phase, the actual program itself, what to do afterwards, shopping lists, and more, so you can track the progress that you've made;

- **Journal Questions**—The list of daily journal questions to help you relax and reflect with plenty of space for you to write your answers;

- **FAQ**—Answers to the most commonly asked questions that I've received on this program; if you have a question, chances are it's been answered in this portion; and

- **Food Log**—A detailed food log so you can track reactions to foods you might be allergic to that might be making you toxic and inflamed;

To download the guide, simply go to:

http://www.ultrametabolismcookbook.com/guide

Join the UltraMetabolism Community Today and Kick-start Your Metabolism

In addition to the downloadable guide, I've put together a special Web site that includes many of the time-saving, program-enhancing tools that the guide has but that also allows you to connect with others on UltraMetabolism.

One of the wonderful things about the Internet is it allows me to stay in touch with many more people than I otherwise could. And at the same time it also allows all of you—people who are going through the same struggles and successes while losing weight and regaining your health—to stay in touch with each other.

When you join the UltraMetabolism community by going to www.ultrawellness.com/um, you'll get access to:

- **Recipe Exchange**—A recipe exchange so you can share your best recipes with others and search for delicious recipes that others have contributed;
- **Message Boards**—Message boards that allow you to connect with others to share advice and tips for getting the most out of the program;
- **Trackers**—An integrated module that allows you to track your health, weight and other vital statistics all online, securely and privately;
- **Private Journal**—A private online journal where you can record your daily thoughts as well as a public blog that you can use to share thoughts with others;
- **Food Log**—A detailed food log so you can track reactions to foods you might be allergic to that might be making you toxic and inflamed;
- **Share Your Success**—A place where you can post your own success story and see and be motivated by the hundreds of success stories posted by others;
- **Weekly Encouragement**—Weekly email reminders during the 7-day program to keep you motivated and on target

To join the UltraMetabolism community, please go to:

www.ultrawellness.com/um

ACKNOWLEDGMENTS

Writing a cookbook is a group activity that includes the farmers who grow the food, the chefs who prepare the food, the recipe tasters who sample the food, and the nutritionists who analyze the food.

I thank all of you.

I also thank all those readers of *UltraMetabolism* who asked for more recipes. Here is your cookbook.

As always, my UltraTeam has helped me in every step of the process: my agent, Richard Pine, who has supported me beyond expectations; my partners Marc Stockman and Jeff Radich, who help make everything I do accessible to so many; Kathie Swift, my anchor and teacher, colleague and partner, who has supported me throughout all the tough corners navigating a better way to care for people with chronic health problems; and my team at The UltraWellness Center, who support me always no matter where I go or how busy I am. Maggie Green and Donna Boland courageously helped me shape the science of nutrition into delicious, satisfying, and healthy meals. You are indispensable. I also thank my fearless helper from Santa Rosa, Spencer Smith, for his amazing attention to detail and for making sure I make sense to everyone.

And a special thank you to David Gilo, my friend, and his family for their endless support, inspiration, and hospitality.

My true gratitude and delight are in having the wonderful team at Simon & Schuster and Scribner behind everything I do—Beth Wareham, Susan Moldow, Rosalind Lippel, Elizabeth Hayes, and Jack Romanos. Thank you, thank you, thank you!

INDEX

Recipes in **bold** are Gluten Free, Dairy Free, and/or Egg Free